A SAFE AND RELIABLE LIFETIME PLAN TO FIGHT ARTHRITIS!

Since its publication nearly a decade ago, *The Arthritis Relief Diet* has helped thousands of arthritis sufferers make positive changes, find relief, and dramatically improve the quality of their lives without relying on medication. Now, Dr. James Scala brings together the most current research about the effect of diet on arthritis in one expanded and authoritative volume. Including useful menu planning tips, *The New Arthritis Relief Diet* will help you discover the arthritis relief measures that fit your unique needs and lifestyle.

THE *NEW* ARTHRITIS RELIEF DIET

DR. JAMES SCALA is the author of the bestselling THE ARTHRITIS RELIEF DIET (Plume) and other health books. He has been involved in nutrition and health research for more than thirty years and has taught nutrition at various universities and medical schools in the United States and abroad.

THE *NEW* ARTHRITIS RELIEF DIET

Proven Steps to Stop Inflammation, Prevent
Joint Damage, Decrease Medication, and
Improve the Quality of Your Life

Dr. James Scala

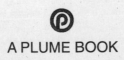

A PLUME BOOK

A NOTE TO THE READER
The ideas, procedures, and suggestions contained in this book are not intended as a substitute for medical treatment by a physician. The reader should regularly consult a physician in matters relating to health.

PLUME
Published by the Penguin Group
Penguin Putnam Inc., 375 Hudson Street,
New York, New York 10014, U.S.A.
Penguin Books Ltd, 27 Wrights Lane,
London W8 5TZ, England
Penguin Books Australia Ltd, Ringwood,
Victoria, Australia
Penguin Books Canada Ltd, 10 Alcorn Avenue,
Toronto, Ontario, Canada M4V 3B2
Penguin Books (N.Z.) Ltd, 182–190 Wairau Road,
Auckland 10, New Zealand

Penguin Books Ltd, Registered Offices:
Harmondsworth, Middlesex, England

Published by Plume, an imprint of Dutton NAL, a member of Penguin Putnam Inc. Original edition published as *The Arthritis Relief Diet.*

First Printing, March, 1998
10 9 8 7 6 5 4 3 2 1

Ⓟ REGISTERED TRADEMARK—MARCA REGISTRADA

LIBRARY OF CONGRESS CATALOGING-IN-PUBLICATION DATA:

Scala, James.
   The new arthritis relief diet : proven steps to stop inflammation, prevent joint damage, decrease medication, and improve the quality of your life / James Scala.
      p.   cm.
   Includes index.
   ISBN 0-452-27951-8 (alk. paper)
   1. Arthritis—Diet therapy.   I. Title.
RC933.S274   1998
616.7′220654—dc21

97-34927
CIP

Printed in the United States of America
Set in New Baskerville
Designed by Leonard Telesca

To Nancy, my wife, partner, and best friend:
Sharing our gifts with others is only eclipsed by the love we share.

Contents

III. Putting Good Intentions into Food   129

IV. Thriving Versus Surviving   201

V. Getting It All Together: People Helping People   269

ACKNOWLEDGMENTS

No book is strictly one person's work, and this one is no exception. A pleasant part of writing this book was the wonderful people I was privileged to work with. They all deserve special recognition for their time, support, and feedback—and my deepest thanks.

Al Zuckerman, my agent: Every time Nancy and I visit with Al we say the same thing: "What a privilege it is to know this man."

Deb Brody: An editor who lets me do it "my way" without pushing, and with much understanding.

Julia Serebrinsky: I can only hope I will get to do another complete book with her fine editing hand at work.

Linda Perigo-Moore: A talented writer and editor who brings sunshine into the day with her kind-spoken words.

The women who have followed this plan: You will know yourselves when you read this book. You made it all come to life by placing your confidence in me. I will always be indebted.

Preface

An Exciting Research Finding

Dr. Jean A. Shapiro and her colleagues at the Fred Hutchinson Cancer Research Center in Seattle, Washington, published a landmark paper in the May 1996 issue of the prestigious medical journal *Epidemiology*. They proved that when people manage their dietary fats, as this book describes, the risk of ever developing arthritis is diminished by over 50 percent.

What makes this finding so important is that not only does the diet in this book bring relief to people with arthritis, as the clinical research proves; it also prevents arthritis in people who are free of it. In other words, if a woman has arthritis and follows the Arthritis Relief Diet, and her children eat as she does, their chances of developing the disease are greatly reduced, if not completely eliminated.

What a gift to give your children! It proves the simple point: Nutrition is preventive medicine, and food is the vehicle of its practice.

Women, Diet, and Health

Biostatisticians confirm that about four women develop rheumatoid arthritis for every man. Taken alone, that doesn't make arthritis a woman's disease, but I think a few other statistics and some personal observations point in that direction. And if you omit from the analysis unique conditions such as ankylosing spondylitis (a rare arthritis of the backbone that affects 10 times more men than women), the female/ male ratio is even larger.

When men *are* diagnosed with rheumatoid arthritis, the disease is seldom as serious as for women. Sure, men get morning stiffness and swollen and aching joints, but the disease is rarely as severely crippling or debilitating for them as it is for women.

Much of this is because of the link between the female hormone estrogen and the development of rheumatoid arthritis. While this link doesn't exclude men completely, it means that severe rheumatoid arthritis is a relatively exclusive disease. You might think of rheumatoid arthritis as a women's club that allows in a few token men to satisfy discriminatory rules.

The exciting news is the scientific confirmation that diet can affect the progress of this disease. Diet does much more than make us fat or thin. I have always been fascinated by nutritionists who, by shifting a few milligrams of a nutrient— not enough to cover the period at the end of this sentence— clear up an illness that had taken the patient to death's door or a debilitated life. They proved Hippocrates' 2,400-year-old advice: "Let food be thy medicine."

A few years ago I witnessed a conversation between two researchers, one a nutritionist and the other a pediatrician. The nutritionist flashed a slide showing the X ray of a child's hand on the screen, on which the physician commented without hesitancy, "That's juvenile rheumatoid arthritis."

The nutritionist flashed a second X ray of a child's hand on the screen.

"A normal hand," the physician immediately remarked.

"They were both the same child, but before and after a nutrient regimen with 50 micrograms of selenium daily as selenomethionine," replied the nutritionist.

The conversation then shifted to a rare childhood disease that occurs in an isolated area of China and responds dramatically to nutrition.

Indeed, my own research on arthritis, high blood pressure,

and Crohn's disease has convinced me that a correctly designed diet, nutrition applied sensibly, and a positive attitude can improve life's quality no matter how devastating the illness or treatment for it.

When I researched a story involving war prisoners after World War II, it was interesting to learn that deprived and orphaned children responded to diet but responded even more when nurturance was added. Combining protein, calories, and the correct nutrients restored the children's health, which had seemed forever lost until the Allies set them free. But the children who also received nurturance—a little love, some positive reinforcement—did markedly better than those who only got the food. This proved a biblical teaching: "Man does not live by bread alone."

Those observations have been reinforced so many times over that they defy my calculus. Modern research confirms that terminal cancer patients gain about 18 months of life by following a course in personal affirmation and motivation. Faced with death, I wonder what I would give for 18 more months. Yet all it takes is a good diet, the right attitude, and some positive support.

In my original arthritis book, *The Arthritis Relief Diet,* I converted the meager nutrition research available in 1986 into a diet plan and enlisted 50 volunteers to test my hypothesis by simply telling friends. Once this group started on a plan, experienced results, and told their friends, the volunteers grew sevenfold.

The Arthritis Relief Diet was a dietary plan anyone could follow because it made sense and used commonly available food. Since then, the book has gone through 14 printings. A week seldom passes that I don't get a call or note from someone who has benefited from the advice in it. Not everyone follows the diet exactly, but each person is doing something positive by taking control of his or her own well-being. So regardless of the outcome, they are all winners.

Ten years after writing *The Arthritis Relief Diet,* many doubters and uninformed physicians still say diet can't help arthritis, in spite of the many published clinical studies proving that arthritis can be managed by diet and that medication can be reduced significantly.

Consequently, I wrote this new edition to include the results of clinical studies that have been done in the last ten years—some of which were undertaken in part as a result of my first book. Their findings are thoroughly discussed in this book and, most important, have been included in this plan.

This book presents a specialized "balanced diet" that eliminates some foods and emphasizes others; the USDA "balanced diet," with its generous use of meat and dairy products, will not work for arthritis relief.

Sadly, the naysayers are usually physicians who don't get the time to read the *Journal of Internal Medicine*; or they are foundation bureaucrats whose agenda is to raise funds; enabling people to help themselves doesn't make the cut. Using diet to relieve pain and swelling seems to undermine the authority of the "professionals." I ask myself, How could professionals *not* encourage patients to do everything possible to improve their own personal condition?

Indeed, you (and hopefully they) will learn in this book what careful double-blind research on supplements and single-blind research on diet has proven: diet and nutrition *can* help arthritis, and even reduce drug use—by 70 percent in typical studies. Reducing prescription drug use is an objective of the medical profession.

All this brings us to a simple point: You've got to eat, so why not select food that will improve your health? Why not adopt dietary habits that will reduce the two most devastating aspects of arthritis, inflammation and joint damage? What's to lose?

A personal objective of mine here is to bring the research together in one place and to explain what we know and how it was learned. I want you to be aware of how much we know, even though more research will always lie ahead.

Another objective is to encourage you to take charge—no matter what your age. By example and teaching, you'll be able to pass the concept on to your loved ones and friends. You'll become a living witness to both personal commitment and the important role of diet.

Finally, suggest to your physician that he or she read this book. Physicians get very little nutrition education in medical school. After all, medicine is a full curriculum that focuses on therapeutic practice, while nutrition is largely preventive medicine. Most doctors don't know this and simply advise their patients to eat a balanced diet. Sometimes they advise them to avoid specific foods when an illness is food based, for example, celiac disease or a specific food allergy. But the nutrition related to arthritis involves all the information in this book, and that puts your doctor in a difficult, if not impossible, situation. Consider that your doctor will spend about seven minutes discussing your illness during an average visit. How could anyone explain the information contained in this book to someone in seven minutes? It simply isn't realistic to expect your doctor to be a rheumatologist, a diet counselor, and an expert in internal medicine at the same time. That is why you have to take control.

A Typical Success Story

Women worldwide have been following this program for years, and some are so elated with their results that they have written to share their good fortune with me. A letter from Mrs. Eve Buckley in the Republic of South Africa exemplifies a response I often receive:

Dear Dr. Scala,

I pray that this letter of thanks reaches you. During June-July 1992, I was diagnosed as having rheumatoid arthritis. Very quickly pain spread from fingers to elbows, knees, feet, neck and chest. I couldn't open a clothespin to hang up my washing, nor open the garage door. Driving soon became almost impossible as I couldn't turn my head and I had to stop knitting and sewing. I live on my own and soon just coping with housework and cooking was more than I could manage. In December I landed in the hospital for bed rest. By this time, I could not climb in or out of the bath!

*Then I discovered your book—*Arthritis: Diet Against It. *I have lived this way now for 3½ years and have no pain. Just my little finger on my right hand will not bend into a fist. In September last year I went to Israel and walked Jerusalem flat.*

I have found that I need to avoid onions, tomatoes, oranges, and grapefruit, but can tolerate three eggs a week and a few new potatoes. I cheat with chocolate every week, but otherwise no cheating—no meat, cheese, cream, sugar, jam, cake, etc. It's just not worth it!

Thank you for your help. And I have passed this on to many others who have also gone out and bought the book. Some say they are not prepared to live without their meat, gravy, and roast potatoes. They keep their pain and deformity. Shame.

By the way, I'm 62 and keep very healthy on this diet. I take three EPA capsules a day and also a multivitamin and mineral prescribed by my doctor. We have lots of fruit in this country and salads, so it's ideal.

Thank you once again.

Mrs. Buckley's letter introduces the basics of the program you will learn about in this book. What's most important is that she succeeded with very little effort. So can you.

The Concept and the Science

The first seven chapters of this book will define arthritis, inflammation, and the diet and food connection—and provide extensive clinical research that proves you can go a long way in controlling your arthritis with food and sensible supplements.

In Part 1 you will learn how diet can help arthritis. It explains:

- Why inflammation is the target.
- How the dietary approach was discovered.
- Why it works.

Approach Part 1 as if you were an explorer making new discoveries. See what scientists have learned and how they have applied their knowledge; then you will be ready to start the diet. Indeed, you can probably design your own plan using these findings as a guide.

Your Foundation for Better Health

In the next seven chapters you will learn that arthritis relief is within your power if you are willing to select food and food supplements sensibly. If you are using medication, you might get by with a little less after you've been on this plan for about three weeks; and after three months, you may be able to reduce it even more. Research has proven that some people will need no medication at all. You will notice less morning stiffness, less inflammation and pain, and more strength. As one woman said, "My rings became loose again." Once your new diet becomes habit, your better health will be routine.

Is This Too Good to Be True?

No! We are not creating miracles here, we are simply applying diet and nutrition to body biochemistry that is well understood. This plan diminishes substances your body produces that cause inflammation, and it increases the substances that reduce inflammation. While inflammation is being checked, the production of other similar substances that cause joint damage will be stopped. So a special diet has a double-barreled advantage: It reduces both inflammation and joint damage. Simply put, this is good science converted into food and sensible food supplements. As my old professor once said, "Nutrition is preventive medicine and food is the vehicle of its practice." We can now include "sensible food supplements," as well.

1

Inflammation Is the Villain

In this chapter we'll review the devastating nature of arthritis. You already know that inflammation is the "villain" because it causes pain, stiffness, and stress and sets in motion the damaging processes that can make a natural marvel—a beautiful joint—ugly, stiff, and just about useless.

A Masterpiece Gets Ruined

Each joint is a natural masterpiece that eclipses even the best engineer's creativity. Joints bear an enormous amount of weight—hundreds of pounds and many times that when you jump just a foot or two, skip rapidly down the stairs, or carry some packages. The pressure on knees, hips, and ankles is often enormous; yet right after jumping, you can glide smoothly across the dance floor and not even be aware of your joints. Similarly, elbows, fingers, and hands can throw a baseball, play a piano, conduct a symphony, thread a needle, and do many other tasks. No robot can do even a fraction of what we take for granted.

We use our joints daily without giving them a thought until something goes wrong. Whoever said the human body is the most marvelous masterpiece ever created grossly understated the obvious. Did you ever give your joints a thought?

What Is a Joint?

A joint is held together by ligaments and tendons—strong, flexible, biological cables that attach muscles to bones. Ligaments and tendons, directed by nerves, allow you to coordinate muscles and move joints in many directions. For example, you can rub your stomach, chew gum, and walk in a circle all at the same time. Similarly, their flexibility first allows our limbs to be twisted, pulled, and compressed and then returns the joint to its normal position. Anyone who's ever sprained an ankle, wrist, or elbow knows both the loss of a joint and the body's miraculous healing power.

At the end of each bone, a firm, rubbery material, called cartilage, cushions it against other bones; so when we step, jump, or just stand still, one bone doesn't actually rub against the other. This cartilage is a natural bushing similar to Teflon (though infinitely better) that protects the bones and allows them to slide smoothly against one another.

Ligaments, tendons, and joints are enclosed in the synovial membrane, a natural sack. This synovial membrane encases the joint and holds nature's lubricant, the synovial fluid, a thin, watery-like lubricant without which the joint would become dry and movement would be impossible. Water is a key nutrient; dehydration, a dangerous condition that affects many parts of the body, is especially damaging to the joints.

What Is Rheumatoid Arthritis?

Arthritis literally means "joint inflammation" and stems from "arth," meaning joint, and "itis," meaning inflammation. Although arthritis usually affects the joints, it can take many forms; some experts say there are about a hundred variations. Rheumatoid arthritis can involve the skin, lymph nodes, heart, lungs, blood, and nervous system; so it can range from a seemingly simple inconvenience, such as swollen knuckles, to an extremely complex chronic illness.

Rheumatoid arthritis can be described as an autoimmune disease; there are two findings that tell us the immune system is involved:

1. During inflammation, white blood cells and antibodies (agents of the immune system) move in large numbers to the synovial membranes that line the joint. These white blood cells and antibodies are attacking the body's own tissue—an "autoimmune" condition.
2. When rheumatoid arthritis is established, the doctor can detect a special protein, the rheumatoid factor (RF) in your blood. This protein is an antibody produced by the immune system.

An antibody is a substance usually produced by our immune system to fight germs or other foreign substances such as proteins. All antibodies are proteins, and RF is no different, except that it acts against other antibodies circulating in the bloodstream. RF only appears in arthritis and its variations, and it is the most definitive factor in a diagnosis.

Hence "automimmune" is the correct term for the disease, and it predicts a devastating outcome if nothing is done. When the membrane tissues are attacked, they counter with rapid growth. Repeated inflammation and rapid tissue growth create an overgrown membrane, similar to a large, internal callus, which ultimately destroys the joint.

As the immune system seems to be in an active though misdirected condition in arthritis, it suggests to many that an infectious agent, possibly a virus, triggers the disease.

A virus is the smallest of all germs and consists almost entirely of protein. It seems that the virus is dormant (think of it as asleep) in the synovial membrane until something happens (usually stress) to start it growing. As it grows, the immune system is mobilized and the joint becomes inflamed, so the attacking cells become confused and go after the body's own tissues as well as the virus; in this case, they attack the inflamed synovial membrane.

Since some people are either more susceptible to the virus or their immune system becomes confused more easily, you can see why rheumatoid arthritis runs in families. There is some concrete evidence that viruses can be passed from one generation to the next.

Women and Rheumatoid Arthritis

Three times as many women get rheumatoid arthritis as men. The vast majority of cases appear between 20 and 70 years of age. If one sex dominates in any disease you don't need a degree in medicine to suspect a hormonal role. And the research suggests there is a subtle but definite hormonal involvement.

Pregnancy

Many women experience relief from rheumatoid arthritis during pregnancy, and symptoms seem to vary with the menstrual cycle. Add to that the observation that nulliparous women (women who have never borne a child) are at greater risk for the disease. Scientists tested this in a study comparing women's number of pregnancies and use of oral contraceptives.

It seems that by not having children, women increase their risk 1.82 times. That is, if you compared large groups of women—let's say two groups of a thousand women, one group that agreed not to have children and one group that had children—and followed them for life, there would be 82 percent more rheumatoid arthritis among the women who didn't have children. That means about 12 women among the childbearing group would be afflicted by rheumatoid arthritis as opposed to about 22 women among the non-childbearing group. While this "thought experiment" would be better if you could follow ten thousand matched pairs of women in each group, it illustrates the difference quite well.

Birth-control Pills

After comparing women who did or did not have children, you might assume that birth-control pills would offer some protection, since they trigger hormonal mechanisms that in some ways resemble pregnancy in women who are not pregnant.

No surprise here. Scientists found that the use of birth-control pills prior to age 35 does indeed protect a woman against rheumatoid arthritis. Again, it is easy to see the magnitude of this effect by following two hypothetical groups of a thousand women for life. One group won't use birth-control pills but will be average: Some will have children and some won't. About 14 women in the average group will get rheumatoid arthritis; only eight women who started birth-control pills before age 35 will get rheumatoid arthritis.

These findings, which I have illustrated by following the hypothetical groups, indicate that there is a clear hormonal relationship and pregnancy is somewhat critical. Yet another study has shown that a woman who decides not to have children and does not use birth-control pills has four times the risk of developing rheumatoid arthritis. So in a group of a thousand such women followed for life, more than 45 would get rheumatoid arthritis!

This discovery led to yet another question: Since rheumatoid arthritis correlates with the hormones, what role does the age of menstruation play in this puzzle? Again, the answer is simple. The older a woman is when she starts menstruating, the more likely she is to get rheumatoid arthritis.

Taken together, all this information leaves little doubt that female hormones are involved. Obviously, there is a serious need for further research. At best, it will take decades to uncover the hormonal relationships to rheumatoid arthritis.

However, at this time we know that the prostaglandins are involved in inflammation. We also know that they can be balanced to prevent inflammation by manipulating omega-3 and omega-6 oils in the diet.

Premenstrual Syndrome (PMS) and the Omega-3 Oils

Gone are the days when doctors said, "Premenstrual stress or discomfort is all in a woman's head." Most medical journals now publish several research papers on PMS annually, which is testimony that it has taken its rightful place among serious illnesses.

Scientists in Denmark, under the direction of Dr. Bernard

Deutch, realized that one common thread in PMS is the prostaglandin PGE-2, which we think of as the "bad" prostaglandin. Deutch reasoned that shifting to the diet this book outlines and using EPA supplements could alter the prostaglandins, reducing the inflammatory prostaglandin to a minimum and elevating the noninflammatory prostaglandin to a maximum.

It is easy to increase the active omega-3 oil, eicosapentaenoic acid, in your diet simply by taking capsules containing EPA. We call EPA capsules "EPA supplements"—just as we refer to vitamin, mineral, and fiber supplements. The sensible use of supplements to elevate dietary nutrients is one benefit of modern food technology.

After three months on the regimen, physical PMS symptoms related to inflammation declined by 50 percent or more, on average. That translates to very little bloating, back pain, cramping, and tiredness; and as an added bonus, emotional symptoms cleared up. It was proved that while the link is still unclear, prostaglandins, hormones, and changes in hormonal levels are somehow interrelated.

What Is PMS?

No two women experience the same symptoms; for instance, one will feel a little tired before her period, and another will become a complete basket case. The most common symptoms include low back pain, cramps, bloating, and an array of emotional problems stemming from depression.

About 70 percent of all women experience at least one of those symptoms between the time of ovulation and the onset of menses, which usually takes place during the last two weeks of the menstrual cycle. Clearly, the onset of PMS at this particular time indicates a hormone-related illness.

Of the many women who get PMS regularly, about 4 percent become so depressed that they can't function properly. They often miss work and become irritable and, in a few cases, suicidal.

PMS isn't brought on by stress or environmental conditions. However, careful studies have proven that a perception of a stressful event will be exaggerated as much as three times during PMS.

What's the Cause?

Medical research is homing in on the causes of PMS, and current literature shows that we can identify and treat the symptoms. Diet is shaping up as a significant factor.

Monthly changes in the levels of two hormones, estrogen and progesterone, are the basis of PMS. Both these hormones decline after ovulation, which in some women triggers the symptoms of PMS.

- A drop in estrogen reduces blood flow to the skin, making you look drawn, dry, pale, and tired. So self-esteem receives a blow.
- A drop in progesterone inhibits the release and absorption of hormones that control fluids and cause fluid retention. So you really are bloated, and your clothes really don't fit.
- A drop in progesterone also triggers the release of prostaglandin PGE-2, the bad prostaglandin, which causes backache and cramping. So the victim really does have backaches and cramps.
- Estrogen decline causes a drop in serotonin, one of several "feel good" brain chemicals. Women who experience PMS show above average changes in serotonin in response to estrogen changes. It simply means that at this time of the month they feel and look more distressed than most women and are, indeed, clinically depressed.

What all this means is that PMS is the body's response to "normal" changes in the female hormones. The reason that some women get it and others don't lies in the magnitude of the changes and individual response to them. It proves that we're all different.

Putting It Together

While some experts still say diet and omega-3 oil supplements can do nothing for arthritis, and some still say that PMS is all in the head, other experts know that diet and PMS are interrelated and that inflammatory diseases all have some involvement with the omega-3:omega-6 oil balance. Some inflammatory diseases also involve the immune system, which, in the case of rheumatoid arthritis, has gone awry. One body of research on arthritis and multiple sclerosis suggests a viral infection can trigger the process.

While these diseases seem unrelated, each depends on the omega-3:omega-6 balance, stress, and hormonal changes. The metabolic similarities are too consistent not to be related and are clearly a fertile area for research.

Many experts feel that some people have a heightened sensitivity to the infectious agent. This hypothesis also helps us understand why arthritis runs in families and affects three women for every man.

If a virus is the trigger, we can understand why arthritis shows up or even flares up under stress, because that's when the immune system is in decline and the virus can start growing; conversely, if a virus isn't involved, why does the immune system in a "suppressed state," such as during pregnancy, start attacking the body's tissues? We can also see why arthritis can show up in children; after all, a virus is a germ that can be caught. It also explains why the new drugs that are used after all else has failed focus on suppressing the immune system.

Similar effects of drugs and diet show the same results for many other inflammatory diseases, including lupus and multiple sclerosis, supporting the experts who link them all together as "autoimmune-inflammatory" diseases. In conclusion, inflammation is the villain, which means that this diet will help these other inflammatory diseases as well. Since inflammation triggers every destructive process in arthritis, it deserves careful consideration.

Inflamed Joints

Arthritis causes the synovial membrane to become inflamed. In addition to causing pain, inflammation limits normal activity, because the membrane becomes stiff and resists movement. Typically, joint pain and stiffness come on so slowly they go unnoticed. You know there's something wrong when you realize the joint hurts and often feels warm and sensitive to the touch. Sometimes the sensitivity gets bad enough that a sharp bump can send you "through the roof." Though the first arthritis symptom usually involves only a single joint, eventually all the joints can be involved. That's why it's often called polyarthritis.

Morning stiffness, the most common early symptom of arthritis, often goes unnoticed until it becomes quite obvious. You wake up and your fingers or a knee might feel stiff and a little swollen; these feelings might even diminish in an hour or so, and you ignore them. Too often these symptoms are dismissed as "I'm getting a little older."

Morning stiffness is a good description, because when rheumatoid arthritis is in its early stages, that is when stiffness and swelling first appear. During the night while you're sleeping, modest swelling of the synovial membrane occurs, causing it to be stiffer than normal. Think of a swollen membrane as the material in an article of clothing you're wearing that becomes bulkier, making it difficult to move; you'd have a hard time at first, but before long you'd be used to it. In the joint, a modest amount of fluid also accumulates, so the immune system cells have a place to go. Therefore, between a slightly thicker synovial membrane and a little more fluid, the joint has become moderately swollen and stiffer while it's been idle.

Once you get moving, the fluid dissipates into the blood, and the membrane swelling subsides; the morning stiffness is gone in an hour or so. However, the joint will be ever so slightly larger, and as Marion, a 50-year-old businesswoman who has followed this plan, said, "One day I realized I was having more trouble getting my rings on."

Antibodies and white blood cells attack the synovial membrane, and it responds by rapid growth. This doesn't seem to matter much at first; however, after repeated attacks and long-term arthritis, excess growth produces a thickened, very convoluted membrane with creases and folds. This condition limits good movement, hurts, and always appears inflamed. Inside, the joint becomes a mass of excess, useless synovial membrane, like an internal callus, with only a fraction of its original use. Outside, it looks swollen, distorted, and sore.

In addition to morning stiffness, lumps beneath the skin—especially around the elbows—often precede the other joint symptoms and are like a warning of impending trouble. Similar lumps and even canker sores often precede attacks in other autoimmune-inflammatory bowel diseases; another similarity that suggests they're connected.

Inflammation, the Target

Leukotrienes, along with prostaglandins, are made from the omega-3 or omega-6 oils. While prostaglandins influence inflammation, the leukotrienes and their byproducts can induce joint damage.

Diet can do a lot to stop inflammation. A prostaglandin and a leukotriene that your body makes from the wrong dietary fats and oils actually cause inflammation and joint damage, respectively. Alternatively, the dietary fats and oils that your body makes in reaction to correct dietary choices do not cause inflammation and joint damage. This theory is the basis of the dietary approach to rheumatoid arthritis relief. You are stopping inflammation naturally when you reduce to an absolute minimum those dietary substances that favor the bad, inflammation-causing prostaglandin and maximize the good, inflammation-suppressing prostaglandin. The same holds true for joint damage, as inflammation and joint damage are intimately connected. If you still require medication after going on the diet, the drugs will work better and your doctor can gain even more control over your illness.

Scientific terms like *prostaglandin* and *leukotriene* can make this plan sound intimidating. In fact, my plan is simple; it boils down to reducing total dietary fat, while completely

avoiding certain fats and increasing others. W
tion of avoiding animal fat, which is difficult
ple, the plan encourages a wide variety of foo
to foods, fats you should increase are availab
plements. This makes the plan as easy as falling off a log.

> Fat management:
> The key to relief

Not Only Joints

Arthritis can affect every part of the body. Rheumatoid arthritis can affect other organs. Vasculitis—inflammation of a blood vessel—causes skin rash, ulcers, migraine headache, and even gangrene in rare cases. Inflammation can involve the lungs, the membrane around the heart, and the nerves. When arthritis affects the eyes and mouth (Sjögren's or Sicca's syndrome), it causes excessive dryness. In addition, there are variations on each one, and they can overlap each other. With every variation, whether it's arthritis in the knees, psoriasis in the skin, or migraine headache, inflammation is the culprit.

More Evidence for Infection and the Immune System

Folk wisdom in Asia and Nordic countries teaches that arthritis relief comes with a starvation period followed by a vegetarian diet. Of course starvation will bring relief because, as you will learn, it reduces the prostaglandin production that causes inflammation and other materials that cause joint damage. However, a person must eat, so how about the vegetarian diet?

Dr. Jens Kjeldsen-Kragh, whose studies you'll read about in chapter 6, has done excellent research on the vegetarian diet. Chapter 6 reviews his proof that a vegetarian diet reduces arthritis inflammation and its complicating symptoms, such as morning stiffness. Most intriguing is his finding that ıs diet alters the intestinal flora, which changes the circulating antibodies and antigens in the blood. These antigens cause the immune system to shift into high gear, which aggravates joint damage, so their decline slows and even stops the joint damage.

An antigen is something that spurs the immune system into action; it can be a germ (virus or bacteria) or a foreign substance such as a protein. Dr. Kjeldsen-Kragh found that normal intestinal flora produces materials (mostly protein) that enter the bloodstream and act as antigens in people with arthritis. He then proved that if he changed the intestinal flora, say with antibiotics or by feeding a culture to people, he also saw changes in the antibodies circulating in the blood.

Dr. Jens Kjeldsen-Kragh's findings take the immune involvement into high-tech research that will continue for decades. What's important here is that these studies help us realize that fiber also has an important role in reducing arthritis flare-ups in addition to proving it's an autoimmune disease. We will return to this point later when I discuss some folk remedies and the need for dietary fiber.

Flare-ups

Over 15 percent of arthritis is not a continuous illness that progresses in a nice, orderly fashion. On a chart, it's like the stock market with its ups and downs, but over time it has a constant upward trend, usually leading to stiffened, deformed joints. Painful periods of inflammation, called flare-ups, last from days to many months. Drugs used during flare-ups focus on stopping inflammation, and milder drugs are often taken in between to prevent flare-ups. During a flare-up, the objective is to stop inflammation and force the arthritis into remission. When the drugs stop inflammation, joint damage may continue, but at a much slower pace.

Flare-ups Invite Quackery
Science Is Your Protection

Arthritis's cyclic nature invites quackery because its flare-ups are self-limiting—in other words, they subside naturally. Flare-ups typically come on from some stress, increase in intensity for a few days, reach a maximum level, and then subside over several more days or even a week or two. Thus, if you did nothing, perhaps used aspirin for the pain, or simply rested a little more, the flare-up would diminish. However, all too often during a flare-up the victim buys a "treatment"—which could range from a pill to an electronic device from a salesperson—that then gets credit for the natural course of events. The selling of the treatment is quackery, even though the salesperson may believe in his or her supposed cure.

Science is your best protection against quackery, because it allows you to witness proof that the remedy it provides actually works. Although for now I want you to take my word that diet works, I will provide proof that it does. When you read chapter 6 you can be the jury and review the excellent methods of the research and its results. Then you will have the freedom to choose that only knowledge can bring.

As you learn about the proof that shows this diet works, I urge you to apply the same standard to every other aspect of your illness. Ask questions of all health care professionals, including your doctor. If he or she can't explain why something works, be skeptical; after all, it's your life. Always ask purveyors of any cures for their credentials and scientific proof of any claims.

Arthritis's cyclical nature makes diet an especially attractive approach because it helps reduce the frequency and magnitude of flare-ups without the side effects of drug intake. If you always take medication when you feel some discomfort, you will be needlessly living with the drug's side effects even when the illness is dormant. In contrast, you have to eat to stay alive, so why not take the opportunity to select food that will improve your health.

Does Stress Bring on Flare-ups?

I have interviewed nearly 375 people who have serious rheumatoid arthritis, and another hundred who have variations ranging from psoriasis to migraine headaches and inflammatory bowel disease. Only one felt that her first major arthritis attack wasn't preceded by some stressful event—but she also pointed out that all the women in her family developed arthritis at her age. Living with such a self-fulfilling prophecy is stressful in and of itself. For others, physical stress, such as a bad fall, serious chill, overwork, and excessive physical activity (to name a few) were most frequently cited as preceding the onset of arthritis. However, internalized mental stress (usually related to family, workplace, or financial problems) is often dismissed by a patient. I remember one person who insisted she saw no relationship between some stressful event to her first bout with arthritis, but when I persisted, she finally confessed to an illicit affair that, because of her strict Roman Catholic upbringing, created incredible inwardly directed stress and anxiety that she couldn't dissipate. The link was established.

Another interesting observation that provides a clue to the links between rheumatoid arthritis and other changes in the body is that a rheumatoid arthritis attack often follows childbirth. It is possible that during pregnancy, all systems undergo major changes, including the immune system, which must accommodate the baby. When the immune system reduces certain of its activities to accommodate the growing baby, a dormant virus in the synovial membranes grows, causing inflammation. Subsequently, after the birth of the baby, a woman's heightened immune system goes into high gear and attacks the virus.

This scenario is only a hypothesis, but it helps us understand the connection between stress and arthritis. In "cold stress" (a more sophisticated way of describing a chill that leads to a runny nose or cold), the first changes we see are a decline in certain antibodies that allow some viruses to grow, causing a cold or flu. Indeed, world-class skiers must train in the cold and frequently they get chills, making them susceptible to colds or flu that, ironically, can ruin their chances in competition. Similarly, the same changes occur with mental, physical, and dietary stress. It all seems to fit a neat pattern that calls for more research. We'll pick this topic up again and explore other indirect evidence.

It won't do you any harm to avoid mental and physical stress. Common sense dictates that it's wise not to get a chill or put yourself in harm's way. Mental stress is no different; it only requires more attention to the things (or people) in your life you can change and those you cannot.

I remember one victim's recollections of how her arthritis first came on: "I fell through the ice," Martha said. "It wasn't a deep pond or anything like that, but it was bone-chilling cold, and I could not seem to get warm until the next morning. Within a week I noticed my knees were swollen." The rest, as we say, is history.

What Do Drugs Do?

Aspirin, possibly the world's oldest and most ubiquitous drug, suppresses inflammation. However, it has side effects that include stomach problems, ringing in the ears, and, with prolonged use, high blood pressure. Newer antiinflammatory drugs (the nonsteroid antiinflammatory category called NSAIDs, which include indomethacin, ibuprofen, and naproxen) suppress inflammation better than aspirin and have milder side effects. The objective in both cases is to stop inflammation and hasten remission.

Arthritis that won't go into remission with NSAIDs calls for "heavy-hitter" remission-inducing drugs such as gold salts, penicillamine, and antimalarial drugs. Heavy-hitter drugs are often taken permanently or for many months and even years to slow (and hopefully stop) inflammation and joint destruction. In chapter 4 you will discover how a leukotriene sets joint damage in motion. For now it's enough to say that the process isn't effectively suppressed by drugs. And specialists must be very careful with these drugs as they have serious— and potentially deadly—side effects.

If the remission-inducing drugs are sufficiently effective, the next step in the battle with rheumatoid arthritis is to stop joint destruction by suppressing the immune process. These drugs, also used in cancer chemotherapy, have numerous, serious side effects and currently represent the "last resort" in arthritis treatment.

Rapid onset or defiant inflammation is often attacked with steroids that can stop the inflammation dead in its tracks. Indeed, sometimes the steroid is injected directly into the inflamed joint, although oral use has become more widely practiced. Physicians prescribe steroids with cautious respect.

In Nutrition, Teamwork Is Essential

Nonsteroid, antiinflammatory drugs (NSAIDs) focus on one process: They stop the production of the "bad" prostaglandin that causes inflammation. Not surprisingly, the natural dietary objective of my plan simply induces the production of the "good" prostaglandin that suppresses inflammation. This approach slows, to a minor (and normal) level, the inflammation-inducing "bad" prostaglandin, and consequently slows, if not stops altogether, joint damage.

It follows that if diet can reduce the inflammatory response to a minimum, drugs can then be used more sparingly, or in lesser intensity, if at all. Fewer and milder drugs mean reduced drug side effects. Either way, the winner is the person who optimizes diet to minimize inflammation. I call it "teamwork in action."

SUGGESTIONS FOR ADDITIONAL READING AND REFERENCES FOR HEALTH-CARE PROFESSIONALS

Deighton, C. M., et al. Rheumatoid arthritis, HLA identity and age at menarche. 1993. *Annals of the Rheumatic Diseases* 52: 522–27.

Deutch, B., et al. Menstrual pain and omega-3 fatty acids. 1995. *European Journal of Clinical Nutrition* 49: 508–27.

Spector, T. D., et al. The pill, parity and rheumatoid arthritis. 1990. *Arthritis and Rheumatism* 33: 782–87.

2

Arthritis and Human Development

There are one hundred variations of arthritis with various similarities and differences; and to make matters more complex, people can have more than one type at a time. Therefore, the permutations and combinations are almost endless.

All forms of arthritis are similar in one respect; they have flare-ups and periods of remission. Flare-ups are periods when the disease is active—joints are inflamed, pain is apparent—and they can last from hours or days to months and even years. Remissions, in contrast, are periods of dormancy when, for all practical purposes, the disease doesn't exist. Periods of flare-ups and remissions vary in length.

My curiosity led me to question the historical aspects of arthritis. Is arthritis a disease of modern times, or has it always existed in one form or another? Does the future look bright or bleak? Will it be eliminated someday?

Osteoarthritis—200 Million Years and Still Going Strong

The University of Kansas Natural History Museum has on display the skeleton of an extinct swimming reptile, the platycarpus, that inhabited the shallow sea that is now the great Midwest two hundred million years ago. All the joints of the left hind limb of this Kansan specimen are deformed by osteoarthritis, and the deformations are similar to those a physician would see in human osteoarthritis today.

Although its animal hosts have changed, osteoarthritis has not changed in over two hundred million years. In the Kansan platycarpus, the joints are deformed by bony overgrowths, and the joint bones contain increased vascular spaces, just like those a physician would see today. This affliction has never changed.

Human History of Osteoarthritis

Our most remote ancestors first roamed the Olduvai Gorge in Africa three million years ago; one million years later, they lived long enough to get osteoarthritis. One million years ago Java man and five hundred thousand years ago Lansing man both got osteoarthritis even though they lived in widely separated times and parts of the world. In fact, had he lived today, one Java man would have been a candidate for a hip replacement.

Archaeologists mistakenly named osteoarthritis "cave gout" because it was so common in skeletons of the cave man. It has been found in the 40,000-year-old skeletons of Neanderthal man; 7,000-year-old mummies from Egypt and Peru; and 3,000-year-old skeletons from the Indian subcontinent.

Here in the United States, excavations of the Mound Builder Indians (circa 850 A.D.) near Port Clinton, Ohio, indicate that most of the adults had some form of osteoarthritis. Burial sites in other areas, ranging from the Southeast in Alabama to the Southwest in New Mexico and north to Alaska, show quite clearly that native Americans got osteoarthritis—it didn't come over with the pilgrims.

Excavations in England prove the pilgrims weren't spared. And not only did the Roman invaders have osteoarthritis, but the Saxons and Celts whom they invaded had it also.

In fact, we all get osteoarthritis to some degree. About 97 percent of people over 65 years old will have some X-ray evidence of osteoarthritis; and 50 percent of these individuals will have evidence that is significant. Unlike rheumatoid arthritis and gout, osteoarthritis is neither a metabolic nor systemic disease; that is, if it occurs in one joint, it does not necessarily spread to others. However, a hereditary tendency apparently exists, and people who get the disease in one joint early in life often develop it in other joints as they age. This is because the cartilage covering the joint bones is hereditarily weak in all joints and more susceptible to damage than average.

Osteoarthritis is the price we pay for living under the influence of gravity. It is simply the wear and tear on the joints, and it can start with an athletic injury, a common household injury, or "just plain living" from day to day. Perhaps in the future, children born in space won't get the disease.

Joint Replacement: Osteoarthritis Today

Today doctors can replace knee, hip, and even finger joints, giving people with osteoarthritis renewed mobility. Most orthopedic surgeons report these "bionic" joints wear out in 10 to 15 years, so they like to put this type of surgery off when people are under age 60. However, scientists continue improving bionic materials to work in better harmony with human tissues; some experts expect that soon they will last over 20 years.

Cartilage Restoration: Osteoarthritis Tomorrow

Osteoarthritis always involves cartilage breakdown. In fact, many cases of severe osteoarthritis are the outcomes of youthful athletic injury to the cartilage of knees or hips.

Now scientists can successfully culture cartilage in the lab from a damaged joint, implant it back into the joint, and restore function. Although this "tissue culture" cartilage replacement is still classified as experimental, it could become routine in less than a decade. The "science fiction" of the 1950s, it will probably be routine before the next millennium is five years old.

Will Diet Help Osteoarthritis?

Yes, the Arthritis Relief Diet and supplement program helps osteoarthritis in two ways.

First, the inflammation in osteoarthritis is identical to rheumatoid arthritis. It involves the same prostaglandins and leukotrienes. Therefore, reducing inflammation is just as important in osteoarthritis as in rheumatoid arthritis. Similarly, the drugs used for osteoarthritis inhibit the enzyme that produces good and bad prostaglandins, so if you can reduce the need for drugs you gain even more.

A second effect of the leukotrienes is the joint damage caused by oxidative reactions. These are prevented (or at least their intensity is reduced) by vitamins C and E, so the same supplement program seen in the Arthritis Relief Diet (400 I.U. of vitamin E and 500 milligrams of vitamin C) should apply.

Glucosamine Sulfate

Glucosamine sulfate supplementation brings some relief to osteoarthritis. Clinical studies have confirmed this, as have people who tried it on their own or at their doctor's or health professional's suggestion. Although it's not a classic herb derived from a plant, you will find it sold in some drugstores, health food stores, and herb shops as a supplement. Ann's letter is typical; she writes from Liberty, Missouri:

> *Dear Dr. Scala,*
>
> *I have had hip pain for years. My doctor is very understanding and has resisted authorizing the hip replacement because it's a little early. However, he told me to go ahead and use the glucosamine sulfate because it would do no harm and he agreed there is a chance it might help. I purchased it at my local "herb store."*
>
> *After two months now, I know it's not in my mind and he agrees. I can spend my day in the store working and then cook dinner when I get home. I don't have the shooting pain ever and I seldom get more than an ache. I haven't used the prescribed "pain" pills and have only used Aleve once or twice in three months.*
>
> *Sincerely,*
> *Ann*

The hypothesis behind glucosamine sulfate is simple: Glucosamine sulfate is the building block of cartilage, similar to the bricks for a foundation. Although I would not expect elevated blood levels of glucosamine to increase some cartilage production, that is what some say is happening. I'm skeptical and believe there is another explanation (not the placebo effect).

Chicken Cartilage—A Future Supplement?

One widely publicized clinical study used a highly purified chicken cartilage with results similar to those expressed in Ann's letter. The researchers, reporting their clinical trial in a scientific journal, admitted that their patient sample was too small for statistically valid conclusions; however, their results were so good that they were proceeding full speed ahead with more extensive research. I am confident this will lead to a new approach to the treatment of this 200-million-year-old disease that none of us can escape if we live long enough.

Rheumatoid Arthritis

Unlike osteoarthritis, rheumatoid arthritis is a disease of the soft tissue, and it doesn't leave a fossil record. Medical archaeologists must search for its evidence among bodies that have been preserved. Consequently, the oldest example of what could pass for rheumatoid arthritis is seen in the 4,700-year-old mummified remains of a Syrian emigrant to Egypt. When this man lived, he suffered with swollen, deformed joints in his hands, knees, and feet. This finding and a few other mummified specimens indicate that rheumatoid arthritis has probably been part of the human condition for about five thousand years.

However, the absence of rheumatoid arthritis in the Old Testament is puzzling. As this disease had such clear, characteristic deformities, one would expect that it was widespread and therefore would have been mentioned in this document.

Probably the earliest written description of rheumatoid arthritis appears in ancient Indian literature from about

1,000 B.C. Caraka, a noted physician of that period, identified and described rheumatoid arthritis as a metabolic disorder that generally involved the joints of fingers, hands, and feet and would spread to all joints. He went even further to describe the involvement of other organs, such as the liver, spleen, lungs, and heart.

Caraka's most important contribution was his identification of gum-guggulu (*commiphora mukul*), a plant derivative that is similar in efficacy to some modern antiinflammatory medications. Besides this remedy, he believed that heat helped relieve the pain that comes with inflammation, so he recommended patients be placed in a pile of fermenting barley, which he concurred was the right temperature for pain relief. He also identified various poultices that brought relief and resemble modern liniments and rubs.

Six hundred years later in Greece, circa 400 B.C., Hippocrates identified and described two distinctive diseases— podagra, which we know as gout, and rheumatoid arthritis. Although these diseases are quite different, they do have similarities, and people can have both together—a fact that created confusion then and still does today.

He described arthritis as a disease that generally appeared in men of about age 35, and he characterized it as beginning in the feet and moving to the hands, where the fingers become slender and cold, which cause the joints to become distorted, enlarged, and progressively difficult to use. And although it was widely used before his time, Hippocrates is generally credited with recommending the chewing of willow bark—an effective source of aspirin—as a means of relieving pain and inflammation.

In 2 A.D., the beginning of the Christian era, Soranus of Ephesus, a descendant and follower of the school of Hippocrates, described rheumatoid arthritis as a chronic, metabolic disease of men in their thirties. In contrast to Hippocrates, Soranus observed that it occasionally occurred in women (especially following childbirth), seldom occurred in children, and occurred in eunuchs (castrated men). Because eunuchs didn't get gout, this was a very important distinction that has no modern parallel. Gout, a joint disease with some similarities to arthritis, is discussed later in this chapter.

Soranus left no doubt that what he described was rheumatoid arthritis, as he accurately described twisted, immovable fingers—often turned sideways—and early morning stiffness. He described the nature of flare-ups, relating them to food, and observed that arthritics could predict the weather. He left little to be said that we don't observe today. But he left us with a mystery.

Why did he call it a disease of men? This doesn't square with today's statistics: three to one women to men. It raises two questions. Was the world so chauvinistic at the time that illness in women didn't count? I doubt it, because a careful study of Soranus' writings proves that he treated women and men equally without bias. Did the disease change? I think so! I suspect that arthritis has changed over the 20 or so centuries since Soranus lived, since there is no doubt that it now affects women much more than men. Quite possibly, if a virus is the cause, it mutated enough to take advantage of the hormonal differences and favors women over men as a host.

The next significant descriptions of rheumatoid arthritis came from Thomas Sydenham, an Englishman, in his extensive treatise of 1676. Under the title "Rheumatism," Sydenham leaves no doubt that rheumatoid arthritis existed; he vividly describes the inflammation, pain, deformities, and suffering. In fact, his descriptions are so accurate they would stand today if rendered in modern English. But this was a full 1,674 years after Soranus! This is a long gap, considering that the disease has such severity and consequences. If only 20 percent of the population experienced arthritis (as it happens today), it couldn't have gone unnoticed for so long. We would have expected to see it in art and sculpture, as well as in the writings of such authors as William Shakespeare.

Why the 1,674-Year Gap?

The first thought is that life expectancy was so short, on average, until the 1600s, that people didn't survive long enough to get the disease. This is simply not so. People often survived past age 40, and the Greek evidence makes it clear that women and children did get the disease. Therefore, life expectancy does not account for the gap.

Some medical scientists speculate that the ancient writings and historical evidence don't deal with rheumatoid arthritis as it exists today, and that what was observed was a complication of gout and osteoarthritis. They argue that because it doesn't appear in writing and art much before the seventeenth century it either got its start or gained new virulence at that time. Indeed, they reason that its absence in the Bible, in art, and the early confusion with gout, coupled with our modern preoccupation with the disease, has caused us to see something in early writings that didn't exist or was no more than a curiosity—a rare occurrence. Clearly, the mummified remains could be a special case of gout with osteoarthritis. These scientists go on to speculate that rheumatoid arthritis evolved from a special form of spondylitis (a type of osteoarthritis of the backbone, which I'll cover later) and therefore it is a disease of the modern era.

Art and Anthropology Give Us Clues

Fifteenth- and sixteenth-century paintings help physicians trace arthritis. Although the painting may have depicted a heroic or romanticized scene, many artists used local people as models and were usually quite accurate in showing their anatomical features. Hence arthritic fingers and knees are shown. In fact, some physicians are convinced that these works of art prove rheumatoid arthritis was well established before Columbus set out on his historic voyage in 1492.

Anthropologists have found evidence of rheumatoid arthritis in several Indian burial sites in North America. North American Indian remains found in what is now Indiana leave little doubt that it existed there before 1500 A.D. Evidence in other burial sites suggests rheumatoid arthritis was present in the New World over two thousand years ago. These findings led some experts to conclude that rheumatoid arthritis was a "New World disease" that was taken back to the Old World by explorers.

However, the fact is quite clear; paintings done between 1430 and 1440 clearly show that arthritis was well established in Europe before Columbus left; and anthropologists have convincing evidence that it was already established in North America when he landed. Therefore, it appears that arthritis did, indeed, develop worldwide and seems to have undergone a sort of worldwide remission until the early fifteenth century.

Rheumatoid Arthritis: Some Speculation

The writings of Caraka in 1000 B.C. and the descriptions of Hippocrates in 400 B.C., perpetuated by Soranus in A.D. 2, leave little doubt in my mind that a form of rheumatoid arthritis existed long before the modern era. That "form" was not as widespread or as prevalent; and possibly it became dormant or died out. Furthermore, if diet was effective in mitigating it, theory would help explain why the disease did not exist among some populations such as Greenlanders or Faero Islanders.

It's my hypothesis that with increasing population, changes in dietary habits, and poor sanitation over the centuries, a new, more virulent form developed. This idea matches that of the writings of Caraka and Hippocrates, who place it as a disease of men, in contrast to modern epidemiology, which proves that arthritis afflicts at least three times more women than men. In support of those who teach that it evolved from spondylitis, we know that men get spondylitis ten to one. The answer is probably lost in the sands of time.

Rheumatoid Arthritis: 1850 to the Present

In 1857, the first illustrated account of rheumatoid arthritis appeared in the medical literature. From then until the early twentieth century, however, a debate continued between physicians who insisted that it was a variation of gout and others who correctly identified it as a disease in its own right.

The advent of the X ray in 1900 permitted physicians to differentiate between osteoarthritis and rheumatoid arthritis;

by 1948, tests were made that identified the rheumatoid factor in blood (RF) on which modern diagnosis rests. Coupled with other blood, tissue, and X ray analyses, RF is the dominant diagnostic factor today.

We also know today that there is a hereditary predisposition to the disease. This doesn't mean that if one of your parents or grandparents had the disease, you will get it; it only means that you are more susceptible. And if it is caused by a virus, then the hereditary tendency is more obvious because of selective sensitivities, selective immunologies, and the subtle differences that make us at once similar and unique.

Is Rheumatoid Arthritis Disappearing?

In 1958, a careful analysis of 1,003 women in England between the ages of 45 and 64 showed that 2.5 percent had definite signs of rheumatoid arthritis. Of the 2.5 percent, fully 6 percent had RF antibodies in their blood—RF doesn't always appear until the disease is in an acute (flare-up) phase.

Compare that with the analysis issued in 1993, when Dr. Tim Spector reported on an identical group and found 1.2 percent had definite signs of rheumatoid arthritis with only 2 percent showing RF antibodies in their blood.

Two conclusions can be derived from this careful, ongoing study: Arthritis is declining, and it is becoming less severe. As you read this book, you can speculate about why this trend is emerging; for now, note these contributing factors:

> *Birth-control pills.* Their regular use helps prevent rheumatoid arthritis; and by some estimates, about 50 percent to 75 percent of women use birth-control pills during their childbearing years. More important, they start taking them when they're young, often around age 15.
>
> *Vaccination.* We know there is a virus involvement in arthritis, and we know that many diseases are now avoided by vaccination and inoculation. Immunization in childhood helps boost the immune system's ability to fight all virus-born illnesses; prevention of diseases like chicken

pox, whooping cough, and measles produces a "halo" effect, an indirect benefit.

Nutrition. In spite of being a seriously overweight world, our nutrition is better. People don't always eat what they should, but by eating more they usually get more nutrients.

Food supplements. Although people don't always take the correct nutritional supplements, they do use more of them, so their nutritional status has improved. Many studies have shown that the immune system, our best line of defense, responds to good nutrition and sensible supplementation.

Gout

A third condition that affects the joints is gout. Named podagra by Hippocrates, it is usually confined to the big toe and the foot, although it sometimes spreads to other areas, especially the thumb and earlobe.

Gout is a hereditary inborn error of metabolism in which the body produces excessive uric acid, the crystals of which accumulate in certain joints, causing intense pain. People with gout should avoid foods that are rich in uric acid, which is found in genetic material. When genetic material is digested uric acid is a major by-product. Foods rich in genetic material include organ meats, such as kidney, liver, spleen, brain; fish roe; and whole fish, such as sardines. Excessive alcoholic beverages also increase the natural uric acid levels, so drinking should be avoided.

Gout appears to have originated with the Semites and is recognized in the Old Testament. Wine drinking was forbidden, and all the sons of Aaron were exposed to a ritual that placed the blood of the sacrificial ram on the big toe, the thumb, and the earlobe in that order—the sites of gout attacks. I believe this ritual identifies gout as a hereditary disorder among the Semites because the ritual was specific for those descendants of Aaron.

Archaeologists identified an Egyptian mummy that had swellings in the foot, and especially in the big toe. Analysis of the toe joint disclosed crystals of uric acid. Because gout was unknown in Egypt at the time, it wasn't surprising that the mummy was of a Syrian emigrant, which verifies the Old Testament ritual.

Hippocrates concluded that gout developed because phlegm and other bad humors accumulated, causing distention of the joint. In his view, its accumulation naturally dropped to the lowest point—the big toe. He also described it as the combined outcome of a rich diet, excessive sexual activity, and sedentary life. In fact, gout comes from the Latin *gutta*, which means "a drop," referring no doubt to the phlegm and humors that Hippocrates identified—dropping to the bottom of the body.

Hippocrates correctly observed that eunuchs, premenopausal women, and prepubertal boys did not get gout. He proposed that castration might be an effective cure. We don't know if his proposal was ever put into action.

The pain of gout is intense; in fact, the old Spanish word for gout also means "screws," because it is like having a torturer put the toe in a screw clamp.

Hippocrates and his followers recognized that diet was effective in controlling gout. His school recommended a diet rich in vegetables, fruit, and fish; no red meats, no organ meat, and no alcohol. Strong attacks were treated with emetics to remove phlegm and bad humors. Sometimes he used "white hellebore" (a very strong purgative) to bring on an attack of dysentery, which, in his words, brought certain relief.

Gout is much more frequent in overweight, sedentary people. It has historically been prevalent among the wealthy—who else could afford the excess meat, wine, and rich food? In Roman times spa treatment began for rich people afflicted with gout, where they visited hot baths while they underwent restriction of meat, alcohol, and excesses in general. Gout was so common in second-century Rome that its sufferers were exempted from paying taxes.

The search for a cure in the sixth century led to the discovery of the plant colchicum, but it was forgotten and rediscovered again in the eighteenth century. Colchicum produces colchicine, which prevents the accumulation of uric acid crystals and is an effective deterrent of attacks.

By the eighteenth century, the medical world understood gout more fully. It was characterized as a man's disease— especially of fat, robust men who had large heads and coarse skin. Attacks could be precipitated by stress, heavy drinking, and rich food. Conversely, in the same people, attacks could be precipitated by the deprivation of food. Colchicine aided the search for the cause of gout; and in 1848, an English physician, Alfred Garrod, developed a urine test that identified people afflicted with gout. He found that when they took colchicine, the factor, later identified as uric acid, didn't appear.

As metabolic biochemistry emerged in the nineteenth and twentieth centuries, drugs were developed that reduce the production of uric acid and dissolve its crystals. Uric acid accumulation can now be stopped at its source, and if gout victims are willing to apply some dietary modifications, they can lead a gout-free life.

Ankylosing Spondylitis: "Homage to a Stiff Man"

When the vertebrae of the spine grow together—fuse—the back becomes stiff. For centuries this condition, called ankylosing spondylitis, has been confused with osteoarthritis. However, it is a distinct disease and has its own etiology. Like osteoarthritis, rheumatoid arthritis, and gout, it has probably always been present, if only to a minor extent.

Nefermaat, the original "stiff man," an Egyptian who lived in 2940 B.C., had a clear case of spondylitis. His spine was essentially a solid block of bone from just below his neck to his rectum. His mummified remains prove that spondylitis has existed for more than five thousand years.

In 1691, physicians described a man whose thoracic vertebrae, adjacent ribs, and lower vertebrae (which are normally separate and distinct) were all joined. Such a man could not bend, stretch, or even breathe deeply—he would truly have been a "stiff man."

Ankylosing spondylitis is distinct from osteoarthritis. During World War II, when men were more routinely X-rayed, spondylitis was recognized as more prevalent than had previously been thought. It appears, however, that the "stiff men" with extensive bone fusion are exceptions. In most cases the disease affects men before age 30, and it is usually self-limiting to the lower vertebrae of the spine.

Some scientists believe that it is an infectious disease with a hereditary tendency. The evidence for this is that men are affected by a ratio of 10 to 1 compared to women, and scientists have identified a tissue type in men who are more prone to getting ankylosing spondylitis. It means that if a man's tissue type corresponds, he has a better chance of getting it than someone with another tissue type.

Systemic Lupus Erythematosus

In 1960, lupus was one of those rare diseases seen by only a few specialists. Very few nonmedical people had ever heard of it. Now, in 1997, most people over the age of 55 have heard of lupus, and many know someone who has it.

Lupus—more specifically, systemic lupus erythematosus, or SLE—means "wolf." It is so named because you can't predict what organ the disease will attack; and the flare-ups are savage, like an attack by wolves.

Lupus is an inflammatory disease of the connective tissue. It can affect the skin, the vital organs, and the joints. It is an autoimmune disease because, as in rheumatoid arthritis, the immune system produces antibodies that attack the tissues. It accounts for the early observations of the Indian physician Caraka that arthritis could spread to the organs.

Eight to 10 women get lupus for every man. Although lupus usually affects the major organs, it often results in an attack on the synovial membranes of the joints, producing a condition similar to but not as severe as rheumatoid arthritis. This situation creates even more confusion.

Other similarities to rheumatoid arthritis include flare-ups and remissions of the inflammatory response, which involve the prostaglandins, the hormonelike substances that can cause or diminish inflammation. And the current hypothesis is that lupus is a virus-induced autoimmune disease. So here again we see that for some reason women are predisposed, a virus is involved, and the inflammatory system has gone awry.

Although I have no more than a few testimonials, I believe this diet plan probably helps lupus. Crystal's story is typical of those who suffer from the disease. Crystal had dealt with the worst of lupus, but she was determined to bring it under control and get off all medication, especially steroids. She stuck tenaciously to this diet and supplement program, kept a careful food diary, and eliminated all foods suspected of causing a flare-up. After about one year, and a very extensive physical—including all the tests—her doctor said it all in one sentence: "I can't find any evidence of lupus right now."

Crystal knows that lupus will always be with her, and she doesn't let down her guard. A she put it: "My guard is this diet and a careful avoidance of all stress."

Over the years since my first book on arthritis was published, I have given the Arthritis Relief Diet to people with lupus. Those who stuck with the program usually lost weight and had fewer and less severe attacks. They became converts. In theory, the diet should help reduce the inflammation and subsequent problems that follow.

Psoriatic Arthritis

As early as 1830, a connection between arthritis and psoriasis was recognized. Psoriasis is a skin disorder that produces scaly patches—usually red—on the scalp, elbows, knees, and neck. Psoriasis is directly related to arthritis and has been given the name psoriatic arthritis. This relationship also accounts for observations made by physicians hundreds of years ago.

About 8 percent of people with psoriasis also show symptoms of arthritis. Like rheumatoid arthritis and lupus, psoriasis is much more common in women than men. And like these other "rheumatic" diseases, it usually appears between the ages of 20 and 30, but it can emerge at any age.

The arthritis of psoriatic arthritis usually appears in one of three forms. Most common is the fingers and toes becoming so swollen that they are called "sausage digits." Next in frequency, psoriatic arthritis affects the end joints of fingers, causing pitted fingernails; it also attacks other joints.

A third type of psoriatic arthritis attacks the spine in "spondylitis," apparently remaining at the base of the spine. Symptoms of this form are the same as ankylosing spondylitis and, in some cases, it actually becomes ankylosing spondylitis. This adds to the confusion.

Heredity plays a role in psoriatic arthritis somewhat similar to the role it plays in rheumatoid arthritis, ankylosing spondylitis, and systemic lupus erythematosus. That is, the genetic marker (a tissue type) can be identified that identifies susceptibility, but it is not a predictor. Thus the implication that a causative agent, such as a virus, and correct circumstances are necessary to trigger one or all of these diseases.

Infectious Arthritis

In contrast to rheumatoid arthritis, infectious arthritis is not chronic; that is, it has a beginning and an end, and it is curable. Infectious arthritis often comes on suddenly because it is caused by an infection—a microorganism is involved—and prompt medical treatment is required to prevent it from spreading to other parts of the body.

Infectious arthritis usually starts as an infection in another part of the body and spreads to a joint, but the infection can also start in the joints. Once the joint is infected, the body's immune defenses spring into action, and inflammation rears its ugly head.

Microorganisms that cause infectious arthritis are varied and include the organisms that cause gonorrhea, staph infections, tuberculosis, and bacteria carried by ticks and mites. German measles and hepatitis viruses as well as some fungi can cause the disease. Just about every part of the world has microorganisms that will cause infectious arthritis.

Treatment of infectious arthritis usually involves antibiotics to eliminate the infection; antiinflammatory medication and pain relievers as required; and rest to stop joint damage and allow the antibiotics to work.

Infectious arthritis illustrates there are many sources of

what is called "arthritis" and that the body's defenses often involve inflammation. The good news is that this form of arthritis has a beginning and an end.

Juvenile Arthritis

Hippocrates first described arthritis as rarely occurring in children. His mere mention indicates that some did exist as early as 400 B.C. Hence, juvenile arthritis has probably been in existence for over three thousand years, like rheumatoid arthritis in adults.

Children get rheumatoid arthritis, ankylosing spondylitis, lupus, and infectious arthritis; and the problems that apply to adults apply to children, except for the resiliency of children. I get the impression that they recover more effectively and more frequently than do adults. However, it is hard to conceive of anything more heartbreaking than a child with one of these dreaded diseases.

Lisa's story summarizes juvenile arthritis. "Childhood stopped when I was five. From then until age 20, I didn't have a day without medication; I don't remember a year without at least one hospital stay." Lisa's arthritis eventually subsided after she started following this diet plan and working with her doctors to reduce medication slowly and carefully. She is happily married and gets along with occasional nonsteroidal antiinflammatory drugs.

People often ask, "Will these dietary concepts help children?" In my opinion, they will, but the clinical studies have been done on adults. The dietary commitment is good at any age and is much healthier than the average diet. The only admonition is to be sure that appropriate supplementation is used to certify that the child receives the RDA for all nutrients. The base level of EPA (see chapter 12) for adults—3 grams—should be the upper limit for children. I recommend strongly that in addition to supplemental EPA, a major effort should be made to use meals to create a good attitude toward the balanced relationship between food and health.

Use food to create a healthy attitude for children.

Additional Thoughts

We recognize that, with the exception of osteoarthritis, inflammatory diseases are probably caused by a virus. Some people are predisposed to getting one or another form, depending on the type of susceptibility. It could be one of several diseases such as ankylosing spondylitis, rheumatoid arthritis, lupus, psoriatic arthritis, multiple sclerosis, or the supreme tragedy—juvenile arthritis. Infectious arthritis can obviously be dealt with by means available today.

Thus I return to dietary intervention. Diet can help—it won't cure—I never said it will. But food is the foundation on which the physician must apply his or her art, and the dietary commitment in this book can be your foundation as you do everything in your power to reclaim and protect your health.

SUGGESTIONS FOR ADDITIONAL READING AND REFERENCES FOR HEALTH-CARE PROFESSIONALS

Dequeker, J., and H. Rico. "Rheumatoid arthritis-like deformities in early sixteenth-century paintings of the Flemish-Dutch school." 1992. *Journal of the American Medical Association* 268: 249–51.

3

"Let Food Be Thy Medicine"

Can Food Help Arthritis?

As Hippocrates said in the fifth century B.C., "Let food be thy medicine." You've got an open mind, or you wouldn't be asking if diet can help arthritis. A questioning mind generates knowledge, so let's start with questions.

Most-asked Questions about Diet Support for Arthritis

I've listed the most typical questions I get when I speak on arthritis or from people who followed the plan in my original arthritis book, *The Arthritis Relief Diet*. If you have other questions, jot them down, and if they aren't answered in this book, write to my address in the back. You will receive an answer!

- Can diet cure arthritis?
- How soon will I experience results?
- What results will I get?
- How do I know it will work? Where's the proof? How soon?
- Does the plan work for everyone?
- Can the same diet work for all types of arthritis?

- How about vegetarians?
- Should I speak to my doctor first? What will my doctor say?
- Do I need to take vitamins? Will herbs help? Other supplements?
- Is an arthritis diet hard to follow?

Can Diet Cure Arthritis?

No! As of now, nothing can cure arthritis, including all modern drugs, herbs, nostrums, and devices! Diet can reduce all of the symptoms by about 70 percent, on average, and 100 percent in many cases. Most important, it can help reduce medication by up to 70 percent, on average, or shift control to a milder drug. This means that many people can stop daily medication and require a less potent drug if an acute attack occurs. That single outcome is reason enough to follow the diet.

What Results Will I Experience?

In a week or so you'll notice inflammation that is not as severe, and a decline in morning stiffness. As one woman put it, "I could start kneeling down in church after about three weeks." Another observed that she could play the piano again after six weeks.

In three months, you will have much more freedom from inflammation, stiffness, and pain. If you've been using an NSAID regularly or even occasionally, you'll need less. As one lady said, "I could ride my bike again, and the Naprosyn bottle never left the medicine cabinet."

You can't see that the damage to your joints is slowing or even stopped because damage occurs gradually, so you've got to have faith that you're building a better future. You're preventing further damage.

You are taking control of your health and consequently your destiny. Not many people take control of their lives, so this accomplishment should really boost your self-esteem.

How Soon for Results?

You'll start feeling a little better within days and definitely in a couple of weeks. However, clinical research proves that when you stick with the program, maximum results take three months. This isn't a long time; I'll explain why.

You didn't get the way you are in a day or two. Chances are you're an adult, and all your life you've been eating a typical diet that contains fats and oils that work against your arthritis. In addition, you have fat reserves that reflect the diet you've been following. Those fat reserves need to make some minor adjustments, and that can take from six to ten weeks. It proves a point about nutrition: Nutrition works in slow motion, and the rewards are worth the effort.

Does the Plan Work for Everyone?

Yes. Anyone who has arthritis or a variation of it will experience some benefit. The sooner you start the diet, the greater the benefit will be, and the less joint damage will occur. So if you developed your arthritis yesterday with some morning stiffness and you start on the diet plan today—you will gain the most benefit. Conversely, if you've had it for 10 years or more, you've already had joint damage that can't be reversed; but that shouldn't stop you from preventing further damage and flare-ups. Let your past experience be a prologue. Focus on a new horizon.

All Types of Arthritis?

Saying "all" is like saying "never." Most types of arthritis will experience beneficial results from this diet plan. I'll go out on a limb and predict that all inflammatory diseases, such as psoriasis, inflammatory bowel disease, and even lupus and others, will gain some relief. Obviously, maximum benefit will go to people with early rheumatoid arthritis because they won't have to go through the suffering that those in more advanced stages have experienced.

Can Vegetarians Follow the Plan?

Vegetarians stand the best chance of success because their dietary habits are "just about there." For example, if vegetarians who use dairy products and eggs will alter fat consumption, and add some supplements—they're well on their way to a better life. As I mentioned earlier, folk wisdom from many cultures teaches that vegetarian diets benefit arthritis. In fact, the best results observed in all the clinical studies were conducted by Dr. Kjeldsen-Kragh of Norway, using a vegetarian diet with omega-3 oil supplements. In part 3 I explain how vegetarians can optimize the benefits of my plan by using selected foods and vegetarian food supplements. We'll even talk about menus.

What Will My Doctor Say?

Medical doctors and the Arthritis Foundation have a tendency to dismiss diet plans with the cliché "just eat a balanced diet." After all, about 85 percent of illnesses will clear up with a standard "balanced" diet, lots of water, and rest. In contrast, population studies from several countries have proven time and again that less than 10 percent of "average people" eat a "balanced" diet. Or conversely, at least 90 percent don't eat a balanced diet, while about 70 percent don't come even close. The diet plan in this book is balanced. But when you have arthritis, the typical "balanced diet" isn't good enough. The dietary objective for you is to reduce some food oils and increase others. A typical balanced diet calls for meat and dairy products that contain those oils. Worse, it allows cooking and salad oils, spreads and shortenings, that have too much of the wrong oils. A slight shift in these eating habits will change everything.

If your doctor says "just eat a balanced diet," point out that the Arthritis Relief Diet is a special plan based on good, solid, medical research. He or she should be delighted that you are doing all you can to help yourself, and you will be an "ideal patient." Your personal diet and lifestyle will have a greater impact on your health than anything else you do on a daily basis.

Should You Ask Your Doctor First?

If you're generally healthy, you really don't need to consult your doctor; after all, the Arthritis Relief Diet is good, balanced food. There are no foods or supplements in this plan that will interact with your medicine or that cannot be eaten if you are allergy-free. If you do have a serious food allergy or sensitivity, you know what to avoid; and that applies to this plan as it does with any other. If your medication can't be used with certain foods or food supplements, you should have been given this information by your doctor, nurse, or pharmacist. If in doubt—always ask your pharmacist.

Will I Need Vitamin Pills?

I use and recommend sensible supplements for everyone. In this case, sensible supplements support the diet and improve its effectiveness. "Sensible" starts with a multiple vitamin-mineral to insure complete nutrition; omega-3 oil supplements (just as have been used in many studies) to enhance the results; and, for many people, a fiber supplement. Several studies indicate that most people consume only 50 percent of the required fiber; and this can affect arthritis. Fiber is essential in the elimination of natural wastes that are sufficiently toxic in your body to cause arthritis inflammation.

In addition, you might benefit from some special food supplements, which I will discuss in later chapters. Most women, regardless of health problems, need more calcium than their diets provide; so in chapter 12 I'll also discuss the research findings on calcium and explain how much you need.

Will Herbs Help?

We are living through an herbal renaissance. People are rediscovering herbs and are using them to replace everything from vitamin pills to the family doctor. By now you know I'm pragmatic and say, "Show me the proof"; in chapter 23 I explain what is known about herbs and why some might work.

Unfortunately, most herbalists are self-appointed experts

who were taught by similar self-proclaimed experts. Ask to see proof of their training and then check out the school they attended. I've learned that more often than not, the expert took a weekend or, at most, a three-week course and received a very high-sounding, pompous degree. It's your life, and if you want to trust your health to just anyone, it's your business—but be informed.

Herbs can't substitute for the Arthritis Relief Plan, and they absolutely do not supply enough nutrients to replace any supplements I recommend.

Is the Diet Plan Hard to Follow?

After reading my first book, *The Arthritis Relief Diet,* people who had been eating red meat five or more times weekly had difficulty because they had to change that habit. However, they were better for the experience, had no complaints, and became the plan's most staunch supporters. I always tell people: "You've got to eat, so why not select food for a more abundant life?"

4

Studies of People
Who Don't Get Arthritis

Every ethnic and cultural diet and lifestyle pattern is actually a field experiment in nutrition. When scientists compare two groups of people with similar genetic backgrounds but markedly different food patterns, they can uncover dietary influences on health. Computer technology has helped make these dietary comparisons possible because it allows scientists to go through enormous amounts of information and compare people who live in diverse locations, while matching them by age, height, weight, and any other pertinent factors. These studies let scientists view cultures as if they were ongoing experiments in nutrition.

Scientists who conduct these population studies are called epidemiologists; I like to call them medical detectives. Their major objective is to discover why an illness is prevalent in one population and not another. Epidemiologists have discovered the causes of cancer; the relationship of salt, weight, and other factors to high blood pressure; the relevance of fat to heart disease; and even that a glass of red wine daily helps you live longer by reducing heart disease. Modern medicine owes much to medical detectives, because they establish differences in diseases among groups of people, and future research is based on this information.

Another use for these scientific findings is in guiding public health. It's an important service to make people aware of the connection between such things as lung cancer and smoking, antioxidants and cancer prevention, and saturated fat and heart disease. Less publicly noteworthy, but especially important to you—such research has uncovered the clues to both prevention and dietary modulation of rheumatoid arthritis.

Comparing Greenlanders to Danes

In 1980, a Scandinavian medical journal published a study that compared Greenlanders to their counterparts in Denmark. Comparing Greenlanders to Danes was no coincidence. They have the same Nordic background with similar genetic make-up, and they form what is called a homogeneous population. Over the centuries, their diets have remained similar in levels of fat but are very different in fat composition. Scientists wanted to learn if the differences in the types of fat eaten had an impact on health. Other dietary components, such as carbohydrates and protein, weren't significantly different, yet another reason the comparison was so important. The senior scientist in this study, Dr. Jorn Dyerberg, emphasized the low heart-disease rate among Greenlanders even though their diet also contained as much fat as most Western countries— including Denmark. This discovery was important because heart disease is the most expensive health problem facing any country. However, along with heart disease, the scientists looked into statistics regarding rheumatoid arthritis and other inflammatory diseases. Their findings were startling.

Inflammatory diseases, especially rheumatoid arthritis, were almost nonexistent among Greenlanders and were much less than 5 percent of what other societies experienced. (Besides rheumatoid arthritis, the other autoimmune, inflammatory diseases studied included psoriasis, asthma, multiple sclerosis, and inflammatory bowel disease.) Though these findings were unexpected from a public health standpoint, they paled in comparison to those regarding heart disease and some types of cancer. Consequently, the publicity surrounding these studies focused on cancer and heart disease.

TABLE 4.1

Relative Health Differences Between Danes and Greenlanders

Disease	Incidence among Danes	Incidence among Greenlanders
Heart attack	XXXXX	X
Stroke	XX	XXXX
Psoriasis	XXXXX	X
Diabetes	XXXXX	None
Asthma	XXXXX	None
Thyroid toxicosis	XXXXX	X
Multiple sclerosis	XXXXX	None
Epilepsy	X	XX
Rheumatoid arthritis	XXXXX	X
Ulcers	XXXXX	XX
Cancer	XXXXX	XXX
Breast cancer	XXXXX	None
Inflammatory bowel disease	XXXX	None

X: a measurable level but very small
XX: definite and consistent signs of the disease
XXX: average occurrence of the disease
XXXX: high incidence of the disease
XXXXX: very high incidence of the disease

Your own experience with arthritis tells you intuitively why experts expected Greenlanders to have as much arthritis as Danes, and possibly more than countries such as the United States. After all, don't your own experiences indicate that extreme cold temperatures and changing weather patterns aggravate arthritis? And that severe cold (cold stress) is enough to trigger flare-ups? Most people with arthritis notice that their hands get puffy and stiff when the weather gets cold. Look at the findings and ask: What protected Greenlanders from rheumatoid arthritis? The answer lies in the difference between omega-3 and omega-6 oils.

A Glossary of 10 Terms about Fat

Although I will repeat often the differences between the omega-3 and omega-6 oils, the following glossary can help you with terms used in this book. People who don't work daily with terms separating fats, oils, and various subgroups—including scientists—tend to get them mixed up. I find that the following 10 terms help me and my colleagues keep them straight. You might also find them helpful.

Fat	Abbreviation	What It Is
1. Fat	None	A food substance that provides 9 calories per gram or 252 per ounce.
2. Hard Fat	None	A fat that is hard at room temperature, such as the "white" fat around beef, or butter.
3. Oil	None	A fat in liquid form at room temperature that provides 9 calories per gram.
4. Fatty Acid	FA	The smallest unit of all fats (and oils). The term "acid" refers to their structure.
5. Saturated Fat or Saturated Fatty Acid	SFA	A fat consisting of fatty acids that have no open (unsaturated) regions. Usually solid at room temperature.
6. Monounsaturated Fatty Acid	MFA	An oil with one open (unsaturated) area on its fatty acids. Heavy liquid at room temperature, such as olive oil.
7. Polyunsaturated Fat or Polyunsaturated Fatty Acid	PUFA	An oil with many open (unsaturated) areas on its fatty acids. Light in color and liquid at room temperature. The more unsaturated, the lighter the liquid.
8. Omega-3 Oil or Omega-3 PUFA	O-3	A PUFA in which the unsaturated areas are in a unique location, the third bond from the omega end.

Fat	Abbreviation	What It Is
9. Omega-6 Oil or Omega-6 PUFA	O-6	A PUFA in which the unsaturated areas are in a unique location, the sixth bond from the omega end.
10. Essential Fatty Acid or Essential Oils	EFA	PUFAs that are essential for human health, if not life itself. We must get some O-3 and O-6 oils in our diet.

Dietary Differences in Greenlanders and Danes

Table 4.2 tells us a great deal about the dietary differences between Greenlanders and Danes.

TABLE 4.2

Dietary Fat Composition

Dietary Fat	Danes	Greenlanders
Percentage of calories from fat	42	39
Percentage of saturated fat	53	23
Percentage of monounsaturated fat	34	58
Percentage of polyunsaturated fat	13	19
Total cholesterol, in milligrams	420	700
Ratio of polyunsaturated to saturated fat	0.2	0.8

Polyunsaturated Fat Intake

	Danes	Greenlanders
Omega-3, in grams	3	14
Omega-6, in grams	10	5
Ratio of omega-6 to omega-3	3.3	0.4

Let's review the features one at a time.

- At 39 and 42 percent, both diets are excessive in fat. These fat levels are similar to those seen in European and North American countries and are becoming common among affluent Asians. It's the result of fast living, fast food, and a shift from Asians' traditional diets.

- Greenlanders eat a diet much more abundant in unsaturated oils (77 percent) compared to Danes (47 percent). The ratio of polyunsaturated to saturated fat makes this difference more obvious.
- Greenlanders eat much more omega-3 oil (14 grams daily) than the Danes (3 grams daily), making the ratio of omega-3 to omega-6 oils about tenfold, at 2.8 versus 0.3. This difference in the omega-3 and omega-6 oils explains the difference in the disease patterns on table 4.1, because omega-3 and omega-6 oils have distinctly different effects on body functions.

Greenlanders' main sources of protein are cold-water fish and marine mammals (whales, sea lions, etc.), which are rich in omega-3 oils and also contain some omega-6 oils. In contrast, the Danes, like many people, get their protein from meat, which is almost exclusively omega-6 oils, although they eat enough fish to get about three grams of omega-3 oils daily. In North America, meat is the major source of protein, and since the cattle are raised on corn, the North American diet is typically low in or devoid of omega-3 oils.

With a few exceptions, people eating a meat-rich diet are in the same or worse situation than the Danes with respect to fat composition. The exceptions are seen in parts of Italy and Greece in the Mediterranean, where there are more monounsaturated oils (MFAs) in the diet, because olive oil is so widely used. People in the seacoast villages of Japan, Canada, and other maritime countries eat more fish than their inland counterparts, and their diets are similarly richer in omega-3 oils and other polyunsaturated oils. However, as overfishing makes fish more expensive, even maritime people switch to meat; and the omega-3 oils are becoming an even smaller part of their diets as well.

If you didn't know about the different oils in the diets of Danes and Greenlanders, you'd expect both of them to have a similarly high rate of heart disease. You might even predict that the Greenlanders would be worse off than the Danes because of their cholesterol intake. Dyerberg and researchers who followed his lead took a careful look at the blood fats of the two groups. After all, diets can be misinterpreted and people can often lie about what they eat; but blood analysis gives a true picture.

By comparing blood and blood-cell composition, scientists learn much about the fat in someone's diet. The fat freely circulating in the blood measures what a person ate recently; the blood-cell fat—the platelets—measures what he's been eating all along.

As an aside, in my own nutrition research from food studies, I learned that each home houses four families:

1. What foods they tell you they eat.
2. What their refrigerator, freezer, and cupboard indicate they eat.
3. What their garbage shows they eat.
4. What a thorough blood analysis proves they eat.

The only definitive proof was what Dyerberg found in the blood and tissue of the Danes and Greenlanders.

Greenlanders and Danes Are What They Eat

Dyerberg's comparison of Danes and Greenlanders was very revealing. Indeed, in the light of subsequent research following these findings, it tells us why there was no inflammatory disease in Greenlanders (or other people who eat lots of fish). Greenlanders eat more fish, which is high in omega-3 fat—and inflammatory disease is rampant in Western societies where people eat less fish, or no fish and more meat. Table 4.3 compares the blood and platelet fats in the Greenlanders and Danes.

Let's analyze the data in Table 4.3.

- Freely circulating blood fat and tissue fat (platelets) were remarkably different in Danes and Greenlanders. Both blood and tissue fat indicate the Danes eat a diet high in omega-6 oils and the Greenlanders eat a diet rich in omega-3 oils. This confirms the diet analysis and proves that the axiom "We are what we eat" applies to Greenlanders and Danes.

TABLE 4.3

Polyunsaturated Fat Composition of Danes and Greenlanders

Oil	Danes		Greenlanders	
	Percentage	Ratio* 0-6/0-3	Percentage	Ratio* 0-6/0-3
		Blood Fat		
Omega-6**	30.7		8.0	
		7.4		0.7
Omega-3***	4.0		11.0	
		Platelets (Tissue Fat)		
Omega-6**	30.3		12.4	
		15.0		0.9
Omega-3***	2.0		13.8	

*The omega-6 total divided by the omega-3 total.
**Omega-6 figure is the sum of linoleic acid and arachidonic acid (AA).
***Omega-3 figure is the sum of EPA and DHA.

- The ratio of omega-6 to omega-3 is very important; it is obtained by simply dividing omega-3 by omega-6.
- The platelet ratio shows a striking difference. In chapter 5 you will learn that these ratios are a telling difference because there is a type of competition that takes place between these oils that either favors or prevents inflammation. The ratio tells us that if an omega-3 oil must compete against an omega-6 oil, it would have an advantage in the Greenlander's body, but about a 15 to 1 disadvantage in the Dane's diet. In short, the Danes have a nominal 15 to 1 disadvantage in arthritis and other inflammatory diseases, while the Greenlanders have an advantage!

Faeroe Islanders Versus Scandinavians

The 18 Faeroe Islands, located in the North Atlantic, are self-ruled; but they have elected representatives in the Danish parliament and are part of the same genetic pool. Comparing them to Scandinavians is like comparing Greenlanders to Danes. The results are very similar.

The comparison between the inflammatory and heart disease rates among the Faeroe Islanders and among the Danes is identical to the Greenlander-Scandinavian comparison. Inflammatory diseases, characterized by rheumatoid arthritis and Crohn's disease, in the islanders are a fraction of those seen in the Danes, even though the dietary comparisons are the same.

Japanese Islanders Versus Seacoast Inhabitants

Japan probably has the world's most homogeneous population. With very little immigration and centuries of isolation, it's safe to conclude that comparing seacoast Japanese to inland villagers eliminates any genetic variations, and the differences observed will have to do with diet and lifestyle. Yet scientists observe the same differences between Japanese seacoast villagers and inland villagers as are seen between Greenlanders and Danes. Even skeptics must take notice.

Since the original studies comparing Danes to Greenlanders, scientists have sought out comparisons where there are reasonably similar ethnic backgrounds with different dietary and lifestyle characteristics. Hence we have learned the following:

- Canadians in maritime provinces, where cold-water fish is a dietary staple, have much less rheumatoid arthritis and inflammatory disease in general.
- Italians who live inland with a diet rich in meat, versus those who live on the seacoast and eat fish, have more rheumatoid arthritis.
- Asians who migrate to the United States and take on our meat-oriented diet, compared to siblings who remain in Asia and eat a more vegetarian and fish-oriented diet, have more rheumatoid arthritis.
- Japanese who live in seacoast villages and eat a diet rich

in fish and almost completely exclude meat have much less rheumatoid arthritis compared to inland villagers who eat meat.

- The most recent research indicates these same patterns hold for multiple sclerosis, which is also an inflammatory autoimmune disease with many similarities to rheumatoid arthritis.

These comparisons bear out the same findings about inflammatory disease that were originally seen in the Dyerberg studies. The magnitude of the differences were not always the same, but the trends were consistent: diet matters.

Consistent Trends Are Important

When parents boast to grandparents that a young child can talk, silence reigns. However, the grandparents catch snatches of speech here and there, and they perceive a trend and know that their grandchild can speak.

Consistent trends in nutrition and health are more important than specific occurrences because a trend indicates a general direction and rules out any chance occurrence. For example, if an illness consistently declines as a dietary change occurs in a population group that remains the same by other criteria, it discloses a direction that transcends any single event. When scientists observe similar disease trends across other boundaries, such as countries, ethnic groups, latitude, and so on, their findings are much stronger.

What Dietary Differences Account for These Findings?

Diet is the main difference in all the population studies. More precisely, it's the difference between omega-3 and omega-6 polyunsaturated fats in the diet. So we need to start by becoming familiar with fats and oils.

Fat is nature's most concentrated energy source. The Danes studied consumed 42 percent, the Greenlanders 39 percent of total calories as fat; that is, both Danes and

Greenlanders get about 40 percent of their energy from fat. This dietary composition is consistent with Europeans, North Americans (U.S., Canada, and Mexico), the British, the Faeroe Islanders, and other populations. Scientists generally recognize that dietary fat energy between 39 and 42 percent is not a large difference. For example, once the diet exceeds about 30 to 35 percent of calories from fat, heart disease and cancer patterns don't increase. To bring about a change in heart disease and cancer, the diet must be below about 25 percent of calories from fat, if general activity patterns are similar. Indeed, until Dr. Dyerberg's findings, it was taken for granted that all such fat levels would have the same disease patterns. How wrong we were!

Greenlanders eat a somewhat unusual diet that includes the meat of marine mammals, such as walrus, sea lions, and whales. Faeroe Islanders eat fish more than mammals; and Japanese seacoasters and Canadian maritime and arctic groups eat only cold-water fish. These eating patterns hold the key to the differences in their disease rates.

Cold-water fish, such as salmon, and marine mammals have fats—actually oils—that are markedly different from those we obtain from beef and other domesticated animals. Although it's dangerous to put "logic" into nature's choice, I'll step out. Fish take on the water temperature where they live, in contrast to warm-blooded animals, which have a constant body temperature. As you know, animal fat is hard and inflexible at room temperature, let alone temperatures of about 50 degrees Fahrenheit or lower. So eating experience tells you that the fats in these fish are different, and a biochemical analysis confirms your taste. And there seems to be some logic in nature's choice: Cold-water fish couldn't move in cold water if they had "warm-temperature" fat as animals do. Indeed, the fish would be like solid blocks!

Greenlanders, Faeroe Islanders, Japanese seacoasters, and so on, eat a diet rich in omega-3 oils (from fish), while most of the world eats a diet rich in omega-6 oils (from meat). The difference was observed in the blood of the Danes and Greenlanders.

As you'll soon learn, one specific omega-6 oil from meat favors inflammation and joint damage, while omega-3 oils suppress inflammation and joint damage. These effects on inflammation aren't direct like medicine; rather, they go through elaborate processes that have only been understood in recent years.

Fish Is Special

Fish has always had a special place in Christian and Eastern religions; so much so that fasting often permits the consumption of fish. The allowance of fish during fasts seems to predate written dietary rules.

Folk wisdom teaches, "Fish is brain food." Although this saying is similarly enmeshed in antiquity, it was revived in the 1920s by Alexander Agassiz, when scientists discovered that fish contained phosphorus, which they felt provided mental energy. They were wrong; phosphorus isn't the essential element involved in this function. But it didn't take long for biochemists to learn that the essential omega-3 fish oils do find their way into the human brain and are critical for mental function, intelligence level (to some extent), and behavior. Although brain food doesn't *seem* related to arthritis, there is a definite link.

Comparisons among vegans (who eat no animal products whatsoever), lacto-ovo vegetarians (who eat dairy products and eggs), and fish-eating vegetarians show they all have lower levels of inflammatory disease when compared to omnivores (people who eat everything). But even more exciting is that vegans and fish-eating vegetarians have the lowest levels of this disease when compared to omnivores.

In addition, vegetarians get omega-3 oils from the numerous vegetables (especially the leafy varieties) they eat and the nuts and seeds (such as walnuts, almonds, pecans, chia seed, and flax seed) that are rich in omega-3 oils. A vegetarian's diet is usually much lower in fat than a meat eater's diet. Therefore, the correct oils (omega-3), though not as abundant in their diet, don't have as much competition with omega-6 oils. More important for our discussion, these diets are also devoid of the one oil, arachidonic acid, that, as we'll see in chapter 5, is critical in causing inflammation.

Vegetarians, especially vegans, have one more thing going for them. A low-fat, nonmeat diet seems to reduce arthritis inflammation and flare-ups in general. This result derives from two sources: red meat seems to aggravate arthritis; and dietary fiber, which only comes from vegetables, definitely helps relieve arthritis.

> The vegetarian diet that permits fish is just about the ideal diet for arthritics.

In chapter 6 we'll discuss clinical studies in which scientists applied this observation in a clinical environment with excellent results. In addition, fish-oil capsules or flax oil (a vegetarian source of EPA) produced excellent arthritis relief.

SUGGESTIONS FOR ADDITIONAL READING AND REFERENCES FOR HEALTH-CARE PROFESSIONALS

Key Scientific Papers

Cathcart, E. S., and W. A. Gonnerman. Fish oil fatty acids and experimental arthritis. 1991. *Rheumatic Diseases Clinicals of North America* 17: 235–42.

Hira, A., et al. "Omega-3 Fatty Acids: Epidemiological and Clinical Aspects." Ch. 5 in *New Protective Roles for Selected Nutrients,* edited by Gene A. Spiller and James Scala, 229–52. New York: Alan R. Liss, 1989.

Horrobin, D. F. Low prevalence of coronary heart disease, psoriasis, asthma, and rheumatoid arthritis in Eskimos: are they caused by high dietary intake of eicosapentaenoic acid, a genetic variation of essential fatty acid metabolism, or a combination of both? 1987. *Medical Hypotheses* 22: 421–28.

Kromann, N., and A. Green. Epidemiological studies in the Upernavik district, Greenland. 1980. *Acta Medica Scandinavia* 208: 401–46.

Recht, L., et al. Hand handicap and rheumatoid arthritis in a fish-eating society (the Faeroe Islands). 1990. *Journal of Internal Medicine* 227: 49–55.

The Basis of Inflammation and Joint Damage

Your body has the ability to make substances called prostaglandins that are either "bad" because they increase inflammation or "good" because they suppress it. Along with the prostaglandins, your body also makes another substance, a leukotriene, that can either cause joint damage or, like the "good" prostaglandin, keep joints healthy. Controlling arthritis inflammation and joint damage by diet requires selecting foods that suppress the bad prostaglandin and leukotriene, and increase the good ones. Effective anti-inflammatory drugs suppress both the bad and good prostaglandins but not the leukotrienes, so even if you take a drug that stops inflammation, joint damage can continue.

Metabolism

Your body is the most complex chemical-processing plant you'll ever see, let alone control. Though not as big as an oil refinery or a food or rocket plant, it's so much more complex, there's no contest.

In a few hours your body can convert a tuna sandwich into body tissues ranging from fingernails (all protein) to muscles (protein, fat, and carbohydrate) to subtle hormones. It can extract the chemical energy locked in fat and sugar more efficiently than your automobile can extract the chemical energy in gasoline or alcohol, which is very similar to fat and carbohydrate. Feel the heat of an automobile engine after it's been running, and notice that it's very much hotter than your body; your body is carrying on the same process more effectively.

Your car uses just one chemical process—it burns gasoline (similar to fat, sugar, and alcohol) to produce carbon dioxide and water while using the energy to power the car. Your body pulls more energy from the same amount of fuel, does it at body temperature, and keeps at least twenty-five thousand other, infinitely more complicated processes going on at the same time; and all the while you don't even notice. For example, while you burn fuel, you also may be reading a book, the print images of which are converted by chemical processes in your eyes into other chemicals that are passed along a nerve as electrical impulses to your brain, which converts these impulses into the information that you see on the page, and stores it as chemicals in your brain to be recalled in some future instant. If that's not marvelous, tell me what is! And that's just a small fraction of what metabolism accomplishes every instant of your life.

Metabolism is really the sum of two parts. First is the breaking down of complex substances (tuna sandwich) into basic components, such as fats, proteins, sugars, vitamins, minerals, and a myriad of other substances. Second is the using of these basic substances to build complex substances (muscles, eyes, the memory storage chemicals in your brain) or to ultimately break them down to carbon dioxide and water for obtaining the energy used for living. Through metabolism, your body extracts substances from food and makes the material it needs to thrive.

Is Metabolism Magic? No! It's All in the Enzymes

Metabolism seemed like magic just a hundred years ago, but now we know it involves the same basic physical laws that govern our universe. It's all made possible by an infinite variety of very complex proteins called enzymes, which catalyze the chemical reactions that convert complex substances into simple substances and extract energy from them that is used to build complex substances. To "catalyze" means to "bring about change without being changed." You could compare it to the official at a marriage ceremony. Two people are brought together for a ritual that initiates their new and marvelous life together; the official who performs the ritual says a few words, perhaps adds a blessing; when it's over, his or her life goes on as usual, while the individuals who got married will never be the same.

Enzymes are very complex proteins that perform their function at body temperature and, like the wedding official, remain unchanged when the job is done. However, they cannot change the direction in which the process goes. That's up to physical laws that factor in "need," which is dictated by the final product and the availability of raw materials. While these physical laws (thermodynamics) determine the direction of metabolism, they don't dictate its speed, or the details of the processes involved.

How your body makes prostaglandins and leukotrienes is a good example of metabolism at work. Your body produces either prostaglandin PGE-2 or PGE-3, depending on the fatty acid available (either arachidonic acid [AA] or eicosapentaenoic acid [EPA]). If AA is in large quantity, PGE-2 is produced; and if EPA is available, PGE-3 is made. However, your body cannot take either prostaglandin and work backward to make fatty acid.

Making Prostaglandins and Leukotrienes

One enzyme group can use two oils to make either the good prostaglandin (PGE-3) and its good leukotriene, or the bad prostaglandin (PGE-2) and its similarly bad leukotriene. Leukotrienes are required for other body processes, so when a prostaglandin is made, a leukotriene is always made at the same time. The body requires both the prostaglandins and leukotrienes to function correctly. Even what we call the bad prostaglandin is necessary in very limited amounts, so it's not all bad outside the context of arthritis. However, the amounts of each prostaglandin produced depend greatly on the amount of each building material. That's where the omega-3 oil, EPA and/or the omega-6 oil, AA, enter the story. Eicosapentaenoic acid (EPA) is converted to the good prostaglandin and leukotriene, while arachidonic acid (AA) is converted to the bad prostaglandin and leukotriene.

This process is illustrated by the following metabolic flow chart. It charts the process much as a road map charts a route. I have oversimplified this chart, but even then it requires careful attention. Let's take it a step at a time, starting on the left side.

The Metabolic Basis of Arthritis Inflammation and Its Relief Through Diet and Supplementation

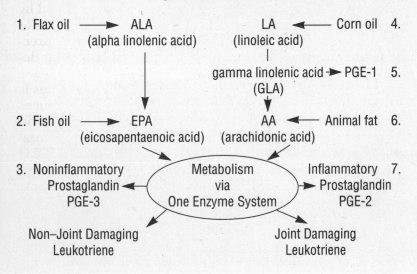

The Biochemical Basis of Arthritis Relief

This metabloic flow chart illustrates how correct food and food-supplement selection can change metabolism to stop inflammation and joint damage caused by arthritis. The objective of the Arthritis Relief Diet is to reduce production of prostaglandin PGE-2 to the minimum necessary for its essential functions, and to increase production of prostaglandin

PGE-3, which does not cause inflammation; similarly for the two corresponding leukotrienes. These changes can be accomplished by sensible food and food-supplement selection.

Each item on this chart is discussed in detail to help you understand how easily it can be put into everyday practice with food and food supplements.

Beginning with the left side of the flow chart:

1. ALA (*Alpha Linolenic Acid*)

ALA is made in the chloroplasts of green plants from another polyunsaturated fatty acid called linoleic acid (shown on the right). Animals can't do this; they can only convert linoleic acid, through a series of steps, into arachidonic acid (AA), which is used to make the antagonistic prostaglandins. ALA is found in all green plants, including green vegetables, leaves, grass, algae, seaweed, and a myriad of others. Mammals, including humans, do not manufacture ALA.

2. ALA to EPA

ALA is important because it is converted to EPA. Fish, algae, plankton, and mammals, including man, convert ALA to EPA through normal metabolism. Fish and sea mammals (e.g., whales, sea lions, etc.) eat the algae and plankton of the sea, accumulating EPA in their oily tissue. We either eat fish and get EPA, or thanks to technology, remove it from the fish and put it in capsules that contain EPA.

Long ago we consumed animals, such as deer, rabbits, and range animals (e.g., buffalo and range-fed cattle) and obtained the EPA that accumulated in the tissues of these animals. Still, you don't get nearly as much EPA from range animals as you do from fish. Fish and sea mammals are the richest sources of EPA because many of them live exclusively on plankton or eat other fish that do. Furthermore, fish also produce more EPA in order to survive in cold ocean temperatures.

3. EPA to PGE-3

EPA is converted to the prostaglandin PGE-3. Not all EPA becomes prostaglandin PGE-3; some is made into another essential oil—docosahexaenoic acid (DHA). Read a label on a bottle of EPA capsules carefully, and you will notice they contain some DHA, which helps the diet because a larger portion of EPA can then be made into prostaglandin PGE-3. DHA in food or from a supplement spares the body making it, so more EPA can be converted to prostaglandin PGE-3.

(A word about DHA is appropriate, even if our focus is on EPA and prostaglandin PGE-3. Docosahexaenoic acid is found in all nerve tissue, including our brain and eyes, where research has proven it is absolutely essential. In young children, it has even been proven to have a role in behavior and intelligence. This is one more reason why this diet program has benefits beyond arthritis and helps all family members.)

EPA Is King of Arthritis Relief

EPA is the critical omega-3 fatty acid pertaining to arthritis since it's the only material our bodies use to make the beneficial prostaglandins and leukotrienes that prevent inflammation and joint damage. Most experts (who have used up to 18 grams of EPA daily in clinical studies) seem to agree that if you eat a diet low in arachidonic acid (found in animal fat), 3 grams of EPA per day from fish and supplements should be adequate; and more is fine.

EPA capsules also contain ALA and DHA, an important combination for another reason—the "push-pull" of metabolism. EPA in the presence of adequate DHA is converted to the beneficial prostaglandins. Although your metabolic machinery will not reverse itself to convert EPA to ALA, having some ALA helps drive EPA to the prostaglandin. Sufficient DHA in the capsule leaves no further need for DHA by the body, and all the EPA is used to make the beneficial prostaglandins or is accumulated in other tissues as required. EPA is also found in the blood, the blood cells, and the walls of blood vessels, where it helps to reduce heart diseases. Although I'm getting a little far afield, it's another reason why the Arthritis Relief Diet is so healthy—a side effect is that it helps prevent heart disease and stroke.

4. Linoleic Acid

Linoleic acid is an essential fatty acid from which your body can make all the omega-6 fatty acids it requires. Since most cooking oils and margarines are made from corn oil, or other PUFA oils, most diets provide an abundance, if not an excess, of linoleic acid.

5. Linoleic Acid (LA) to Gamma Linolenic Acid (GLA)

Linoleic acid is converted to many other fatty acids, including a transitory, short-lived material called gamma linolenic acid (GLA), another omega-6 oil. By "transitory" and "short-lived," we mean that GLA is not available in quantity because it is used about as quickly as it is made. However, under some circumstances, very little, if any, is made. A circumstance under which GLA isn't made arises when an abundance of AA causes "feedback inhibition." This simply means that there is no need for the body to make AA, so the LA to AA system simply shuts down.

6. Gamma Linolenic Acid (GLA) and Prostaglandin PGE-1

We get very little GLA in our diet, as it is a seed oil only found most abundantly in evening primrose and black currant seeds, which are impractical dietary sources. Metabolism converts some GLA to prostaglandin PGE-1. Most researchers recognize that PGE-1 modulates the inflammation caused by PGE-2 when AA is available in modest quantities. Your body can only produce PGE-1 in very minor quantities; consequently, when dietary AA is abundant, the body produces excessive PGE-2, and any beneficial effect of PGE-1 is lost.

7. Gamma Linolenic Acid (GLA) to Arachidonic Acid (AA)

GLA is generally considered an "intermediate" between linoleic acid (LA) and AA. Our body needs: (1) both GLA and LA; (2) some AA; and (3) the prostaglandin PGE-2.

However, when the diet provides excess AA, too much PGE-2 is produced, and the AA swamps the small amount of EPA that is converted by the same enzyme system. A diet rich in AA also renders the small amount of prostaglandin PGE-1 useless.

One more time: A diet rich in animal foods and baked goods made with animal fat (e.g., butter) is excessive in arachidonic acid and favors inflammation.

Stopping Arthritis Inflammation and Joint Damage

The metabolic flow chart illustrates how correct food and food supplement selection can change metabolism to stop inflammation and joint damage. The following six steps are essential in controlling arthritis inflammation and joint damage:

1. Eliminate animal foods—arachidonic acid. This will normalize prostaglandin PGE-2 production.
2. Obtain dietary EPA by eating cold-water fish as your protein source. This will favor prostaglandin PGE-3.
3. Cooking and salad oils: select oils rich in ALA, such as canola oil, to favor natural EPA production.
4. Use flax oil: add it sensibly to food, such as salads and cereals, to favor natural EPA and prostaglandin PGE-3. Do not fry or bake with flax oil. Take up to 30 grams of flax oil in capsules, or add it, in liquid form, to food.
5. Sensible EPA supplementation: take three grams of EPA daily (over nine grams daily is safe), or take less EPA (e.g., two grams) with 15 grams of flax oil.
6. Sensible GLA supplementation: take evening primrose or borage oil supplements (one gram daily) in moderation to favor prostaglandin PGE-1, which modulates the inflammatory effect of prostaglandin PGE-2.

Nothing's Perfect

A serious problem pops up in your metabolism of linoleic acid. Specifically, your body seems equipped to work best in a food environment which is abundant in the omega-3 oils, including ALA and EPA, with limited amounts of the omega-6 oils, LA and especially AA. Since the body expects an abundance of the omega-3 oils, it has a much better affinity for the omega-6 oils, which are expected to be scarce. Our dietary system has completely turned that system upside down, because we eat foods generally rich in the omega-6 oils and totally lacking in the omega-3 oils. For many people this is not a problem, but it's a disaster for people with any inflammatory disease.

A Flaw in the System; EPA Versus AA

Now you can visualize your problem. The enzyme that catalyzes EPA into the good prostaglandin PGE-3 and the good leukotriene works better (scientists say, has a better "affinity") with AA because throughout most of human history AA has been scarce. Look at it as a "natural choice" prejudiced by evolution, as directed by the Creator.

This means that if there is an equal amount of AA and EPA available to the enzyme, it would take AA and make prostaglandin PGE-2, leaving EPA sitting on the sideline. So a diet that supplies a lot of AA and little EPA is predisposed to make only the bad prostaglandin and leukotriene. Worse yet, the average diet is so overly excessive in animal fat that the enzyme never sees EPA, and only prostaglandin PGE-2 is made.

The abundance of AA causes another flaw to emerge— the production of PGE-1 is stopped, as I mentioned already. While PGE-1 can't substitute for PGE-2 or PGE-3, it can help modulate some of the inflammation caused by PGE-2. However, in a diet rich in AA, PGE-1 is not made.

> YOU WANT:
> MORE EPA
> LESS AA

The opposite happens in a diet with more EPA than AA— such as the diets of Greenlanders, seacoast villagers in many countries, or vegetarians. In these diets, the good prostaglandin and leukotriene dominate, because EPA is abundant. However, since the enzyme has a greater affinity for AA, prostaglandin PGE-2 is made in sufficient amounts for its essential functions. Thus there's no inflammation and joint damage among people who have a diet rich in EPA. It's not magic, it's simply normal metabolism.

Why Would the Enzyme Prefer AA?

Your body's enzymes reflect the food environment in which our species developed. Just a few hundred years ago, let alone one thousand or ten thousand years or more, alpha linoleic acid (ALA), eicosapentaenoic acid (EPA) and docosahexaenoic acid (DHA) were plentiful in the foods our ancestors ate. Salads were made from purslane, a vegetable rich in ALA. Range animals fed on grasses that were rich in ALA, so their meat was limited in arachidonic acid (AA) and rich in ALA, EPA, and DHA; the same was true for rabbits and other small game animals.

In contrast, linoleic acid (LA) was not very abundant, and AA was quite scarce because it's strictly an animal material. After all, for much of our history we were mostly vegetarian, and our meat was game, which contains EPA and AA. Farm animals in those times ate grass and straw—not corn, which was a New World food. With these omega-3 oils in abundance, the enzyme served our needs well, because AA was scarce in our diet and it is necessary for the prostaglandin PGE-2. Hence, the enzyme working more efficiently on AA than it does on EPA only reflects the conditions of our early environment. By favoring AA, a scarce material was converted to a material needed in limited quantity. This is just another example of the efficiency of the human body and how slowly we change.

This enzyme preference for AA suggests that there is a logic to evolution—or, better still, the hand of God favored a more modest diet. Both interpretations are correct. Evolution's logic is survival and the ability to thrive. Or if you prefer the hand of God, the same conclusion applies, as our ability to thrive and control our environment is obvious, even if you take issue with what we've done to it.

Once again, balance plays an important role in the metabolic picture. When PGE-2 is produced in minor quantities, the other prostaglandin PGE-1, similarly produced in limited quantities, seems to balance PGE-2's inflammatory impact. However, since PGE-1 is produced in very limited quantities, a food environment that provides excess AA will never provide enough PGE-1. Worse yet, when dietary AA is available, the production of PGE-1 stops, suggesting a sort of metabolic traffic jam.

A System Gone Wrong

If you have arthritis and your diet favors the wrong foods, you probably take drugs that suppress PGE-3 but also prevent PGE-2 production. So while you diminish the inflammation, you actually cause long-term problems. It's instructive to consider each factor.

First, a diet that has been excessive in animal fat has created fat reserves high in AA. Add to those fat reserves a continuous dietary supply of AA, and the dominant (if not only) prostaglandin produced is PGE-2. Therefore, inflammation is favored, and its accompanying leukotriene continues to favor joint damage.

Second, while PGE-1 seems to suppress the inflammation caused by PGE-2, it really works in an environment where there is little PGE-2, not one in which it dominates. To make matters worse, there are no common dietary sources of gamma linolenic acid (GLA) from which PGE-1 is made, so only very small amounts are produced naturally by the body. As we will see in chapter 7, when GLA is taken as a supplement, it seems to suppress inflammation.

Third, a diet rich in AA cannot possibly also supply enough EPA to produce prostaglandin PGE-3. This means the prostaglandin-producing enzyme system will continue making large quantities of PGE-2 and no PGE-3. If that's not bad enough, the use of typical NSAIDs (nonsteroid anti-inflammatory drugs) makes matters worse.

Fourth, when NSAIDs are used in this dietary environment, they suppress the inflammation by stopping PGE-3 and bring relief to the victim, but they also precipitate other problems. For while NSAIDs prevent PGE-3, they don't stop leukotriene production. There is one bit of good news, however. Although leukotriene production does cause some joint damage, it is probably suppressed by the general slow-down of prostaglandin production.

This is where metabolic maps resemble roads. It's as if a bridge is jammed, causing tie-ups in all the peripheral roads so that nothing moves. Sticking with the "road map" and clogged intersections analogy, we can summarize the following diet design:

- Aggressively minimize dietary AA to stop excess PGE-2.
- Moderate dietary linoleic acid to support natural PGE-2 levels and natural PGE-1.
- Aggressively increase dietary ALA and EPA.
- Use EPA and/or ALA supplements sensibly to favor PGE-3.
- Use GLA supplements sensibly to make PGE-1.
- Make sure your diet plan is abundant in vegetable foods and provides dietary fiber.

If we put these points to work correctly, the dietary program will increase EPA naturally, elevate the good prostaglandins, and diminish the bad prostaglandins, as the clinical studies have verified.

6

Clinical Results

Numerous studies have proved that arthritis can be controlled by diet, and such evidence can help you make an informed choice regarding your treatment.

- Double-blind clinical studies have proved that eicosapentaenoic acid (EPA) significantly improves rheumatoid arthritis. (A double-blind study is an experimental testing procedure in which neither the researcher nor the subjects know who is receiving the substance or treatment being studied.)
- Single-blind studies that used double-blind EPA supplements within the diet proved that diet and supplements together improve arthritis even more than EPA supplements alone. (A single-blind study is an experimental procedure in which the experimenters know the composition of the test and control groups but the subjects do not.)
- Other studies focused on discovering which foods can cause arthritic flare-ups.

The information in this chapter will answer some of the questions you have about using diet to control your arthritis, and it should make you feel comfortable about doing so. Share this information with your doctor.

Here are some of the common questions:

How and why are dietary and supplement studies conducted?

What results did the EPA supplement studies produce?

What results did diet studies show?

How long did it take for the results to be observed?

Does food influence arthritis flare-ups?

How can these findings help me?

Why Clinical Studies?

Up to now, we've studied—through the eyes of epidemiologists—populations that don't get rheumatoid arthritis. I've explored with you the metabolism that could explain these excellent scientific observations, and I have outlined a dietary program. Shouldn't I put it to the test? After all, isn't this what I recommend for everyone in the first chapter? This is where clinical studies enter the picture.

No matter how good our knowledge of nutrition, biochemistry, and metabolism, our hypothesis must be tested. Scientific testing is essential. The human body is not only complex, but too often it can surprise us with unexpected shifts. That is why we do clinical studies—to rule out flaws in our thinking and to uncover the unexpected.

Double-Blind: Avoiding the Placebo Effect

Any results from a clinical test can be influenced by the attitudes of clinicians, assistants, and patients, not to mention the volunteers with arthritis. We call this influence the placebo effect, and it can be as much as a 15 percent effect, where arthritis seems to improve no matter what's done. In other words, 15 percent of the participants could do significantly better even if you just gave them a starch pill, called a placebo. A placebo is given because scientists recognize that attitude can produce either improvement or failure (although it's usually improvement). Think about research objectives for a moment and you'll get the point.

For example, a researcher reviews the scientific findings discussed in the first chapters of this book and develops a hypothesis about the omega-3 oils and arthritis relief. The scientist then writes a carefully thought-out research proposal to test the hypothesis in a clinical study. He or she believes the omega-3 oils will improve arthritis and sets out to prove it. With the urgent needs in clinical medicine and competition for scarce resources, researchers can't afford time proving a negative. Hence, research scientists are aiming to prove their ideals; so their attitudes have to be positive.

Second, the arthritic volunteer looks to improve his or her life through a new treatment, and hopes that the sacrifice of being a guinea pig will help other similarly afflicted people. Consequently, positive attitude contributes to a personal desire to get better and to help others.

Now add a close working relationship between the clinician and the patient volunteer, who might see one or more staff members weekly, if not every few days. Enthusiasm is infectious, and everyone's spirits lift as they always do around positive people. Add the fact that most people with a chronic illness never get involved in seeking a cure.

It all adds up to a simple point: everyone in the study is pulling hard for good results. If studies aren't carefully designed, a 15 percent change will be observed no matter what; rarely, if ever, does change go in the negative direction.

Double-blind studies eliminate the placebo effect. This safeguard simply insures that the patient doesn't know whether she's getting the real thing (in this case, the omega-3 oil) or a placebo. Nor does the researcher know which patient is getting the oil. An accountant or similarly uninvolved person codes the materials, locks the code in a safe, and releases it only after all the results are tabulated by a diassociated statistician. Scientists can then compare results against the actual material used.

Crossover Studies: Each Person Is a Control

Another approach, often used in food-related studies, is a crossover design. This variation means that each patient will get both the real omega-3 oil and a placebo—at different times in a random order among volunteers. For example, some patients get omega-3 oil for three months while others get a placebo pill; a "washout" period follows, when all the patients take nothing and follow a similar diet; then the supplements are reversed. Hence this crossover study is also double-blind, providing comparisons between patients, but it has the added value that each patient acts as his or her own control.

Time is a disadvantage in the crossover design, because it's difficult to keep a study going for six to twelve months. After all, the patients must be able to alter their lives sufficiently so that they can come to the clinic, and submit to blood tests and physical evaluations. In addition, the longer the study, the greater its cost, so there's a financial consideration as well. However, it's a superb method, since the crossover design eliminates a variable that has emerged in some arthritis studies. EPA creates a somewhat fishy aftertaste in some people because of normal variations in the muscle that closes the stomach. This means that some people will know when they're getting something "fishy." The crossover design is the best way to rule out this "guessing game."

Single-Blind: Dietary Studies Can't Be Double-Blind

A necessary variation in dietary studies is the "single-blind" technique. Face it, a diet that contains fish or is vegetarian, as compared to, say, meat or poultry, is obvious to those who do the eating, let alone to the people who do the cooking and serving. Indeed, if you were blindfolded, you could tell whether or not you were eating some variety of fish, rather than beef or turkey. Therefore, scientists must use the single-blind approach in most dietary studies.

A single-blind study usually means the patient knows his diet is different even if he's getting a daily pill that is double-blinded. However, even if the patient is aware of the diet, it can still be hidden from the clinician who is evaluating the results. After all, the clinician only examines the patient's physical changes and never sees what he eats. Furthermore, clinicians can avoid discussing food at all and can stick to "Does this hurt?" and so on.

For example, suppose the criteria for the experiment are morning stiffness and grip strength. The clinician testing either or both of those criteria and the technicians taking and analyzing blood don't need to know what a patient is eating. In fact, they can be recruited outside the study as evaluators and instructed to only discuss symptoms. In this way, single-blind dietary studies are completely objective with no placebo effect.

A Personal Experience

While visiting a study conducted by Dr. Tony Albanese, a pioneer in osteoporosis research, I asked the X-ray technician how the study was going. Her reply was: "I can tell you who's getting the real thing and who's on the placebo."

"How?" I asked, knowing that all she did was conduct a bone density scan.

"I'm supposed to note, in their words, how everything is going when they come in here," she replied. "If they have any serious problems, I'm to send them to the administrator."

"And what do they tell you?" I asked.

"Well, there's clearly one group that has more energy, goes to the movies more, claims they're eating more and even gaining weight. I'll bet a day's pay I can tell you exactly who is on the test material." I took her up on the bet.

The study was using calcium in a multivitamin matrix to restore bone density. One group received a starch placebo with no extra vitamins or calcium, and the other group got the real thing. When the study was finished, she was correct down to every person; and she got an extra day's pay!

The technician's observation produced an unexpected result. When elderly people, like anyone else, receive complete nutrition, their energy improves, their appetite increases, and they become sharper and more active. There was no way these results could be "blinded" out of this particular study; but the X rays told the real story about bone changes, so attitudes didn't matter much. Dr. Albanese's studies have since been confirmed all over the world.

The Results

I have reviewed 13 major clinical studies conducted and published between 1985 and 1995 and summarized their double-blind crossover results in Table 6.1. Medical references are listed at the end of the chapter.

TABLE **6.1**

A Summary of Clinical Research on Rheumatoid Arthritis

Amount of Omega-3 Oil (Grams/day)	Duration (Weeks)	Clinical Measurements	Principal Investigator*
3.0	12	Number of tender joints (decreased) Morning stiffness (decreased)	Kremer, J.M. (1)
4.5	14	Number of tender joints (decreased) Morning stiffness (decreased) Time to fatigue (lengthened) Blood chemistry (improved)	Kremer, J.M. (2)
3.2 & 6.4	24	Number of tender joints (decreased) Number of swollen joints (decreased) Morning stiffness (decreased) Grip strength (increased) Blood chemistry (improved)	Kremer, J. M. (3)
2.7	4	Ritchie Joint Index (improved) Morning stiffness (decreased) Grip strength (increased)	Magaro, M. (4)
0.5	52	Daily intake NSAID (decreased)	Belch, J. J. F. (5)
5.2	12	Number of tender joints (decreased) Grip strength (increased) Blood chemistry (improved)	Cleland, L. G. (6)

Amount of Omega-3 Oil (Grams/day)	Duration (Weeks)	Clinical Measurements	Principal Investigator*
3.4	12	Number of tender joints (decreased) Morning stiffness (decreased) Blood chemistry (improved)	van der Temple, H. (7)
3.0	26	Global assessment (improved) NSAID requirement (decreased)	Sköldstam, L. (8)
5.0	16	Morning stiffness (decreased)	Kjeldsen-Kragh, J. (9)
3.6	12	Number of tender joints (decreased) Morning stiffness (decreased)	Nielsen, G. L. (10)
130 mg/kg body weight (e.g., 9.1 grams/day @ 150 lbs.)	30	Number of tender joints (decreased) Morning stiffness (decreased) Global assessment (improved) After stopping NSAIDs, improvement continued	Kremer, J. M. (11)
2.6 & 1.3	52	Global assessment (improved) NSAID requirement (decreased) (2.6 grams/day only)	Geusens, P. (12)
2.8	52	NSAID requirement (decreased) (No NSAIDs needed after EPA stopped)	Lau, C. S. (13)

*Numbers in parentheses refer to the studies listed at the end of this chapter.

Included in Table 6.1 are the grams of omega-3 (EPA) given as supplements per day. Best results appear to occur with between 3 and 5 grams of EPA daily, which is about the level used in Kremer's study published in 1995. Kremer and his coworkers used 130 milligrams per kilogram of body weight, which comes to just under 60 milligrams per pound;

so five grams would be enough for a 100-pound person and 10 grams enough for a 200-pound person. If you commit to the Arthritis Relief Diet, about three grams will be adequate if you weigh 100 pounds (6 for 200 pounds).

In these studies just about every clinical arthritis criterion improved. Consider each as it could relate to your own future well-being. The subjects reported, and the clinicians confirmed by appropriate tests, the following results:

1. *Number of tender joints decreased consistently.* You could expect that your joints will not hurt as much—and joint damage would diminish proportionately.
2. *Morning stiffness improved consistently.* Simply put, you will wake up with your joints being more flexible and able to move without pain. A side effect not evaluated in this test was swelling, which also decreased.
3. *Time to fatigue lengthened.* You will go much longer during the day without feeling tired; notice that you have more energy; and probably experience a more positive outlook.
4. *Grip strength improved.* Your ability to squeeze calipers will increase; this is a completely objective measure. Practically, it means that daily tasks, such as picking up a coffee cup, pumping gasoline, or anything calling for dexterity, become easier. Grip strength confirms a decline in inflammation and proves that tendons and muscles are functioning better.
5. *Daily use of NSAIDs declined.* You will not need as much medication on average. Since this result was about 70 percent successful in the study, it means some people will be able to eliminate NSAIDs altogether. Since all drugs have unwanted side effects, even a modest reduction in the drug dosage means this dietary approach would be more than worthwhile.
6. *Ritchie Joint Index improved.* This means that a combination of joint stiffness and grip strength will improve. The Ritchie Index is a more quantitative measure than other measures.
7. *Global assessment improved.* The clinical expert's general assessment of all criteria improved in the subjects. To

the average person, what this means is you'll notice yourself saying, "I feel better."

8. *Biochemical changes improved.* This means that the flow chart in chapter 5 changed as predicted. Prostaglandin PGE-3 and the good leukotriene increased, while the bad prostaglandin and bad leukotriene deceased. These biochemical measures would be valid even if the studies were not double-blinded, because they couldn't be influenced by attitude.

Taken together, these clinical results confirm that the observations described in chapters 1 and 4 are the result of diet and not some other factor. They confirm that the metabolic reasoning discussed in chapter 5 is correct.

To you they have a simple meaning: You can eat correctly to improve your arthritis. In addition, the sensible use of EPA and flax oil supplements can add to the positive dietary effects. Now let's consider some realistic aspects.

Nutrition Works in Slow Motion

Although the clinical studies were spectacular, they proved that it takes about 12 weeks for complete results to emerge; so you have to make a serious commitment, and have confidence that you will achieve the desired results. They also left your part undone, which is diet.

Most of the clinical studies used either three or six grams daily of EPA omega-3 oil supplements. Indeed, the dose-response relationship was further confirmation that the supplements work. This proves that diet combined with sensible EPA and flax oil supplements is the best way to manage arthritis.

Studies that Combine Diet and EPA Supplements

Oriental and Nordic folk wisdom teaches that arthritis yields to a vegetarian diet. Indeed, this centuries-old folk wisdom is much like the Greenlanders' versus the Danes' experience. If just a few people followed a vegetarian diet, the results would be merely interesting. However, when the wisdom (or more accurately, the teaching) survives centuries, it becomes an ongoing experiment; and it deserves critical study. Besides, it makes sense in view of chapter 5 and the flow chart.

Dr. Jens Kjeldsen-Kragh, a Norwegian research physician, has put the vegetarian approach to several such tests. In the simplest approach, he had two groups undergo a "washout" period in a health spa, then put one group on a vegetarian diet and the other on a regular, nonrestricted diet.

A vegetarian diet reduces dietary arachidonic acid (AA), so your body will naturally make the small amount required for good health. And if a vegetarian diet is well designed, it will include alpha linolenic acid (ALA) and EPA so your body can make significant amounts of the good prostaglandin and leukotriene. Can you guess what the second variation was?

It was to supplement the vegetarian diet with omega-3 oils, specifically EPA. This second design includes the best of both possibilities, because it insures the critical enzyme will get much more EPA than AA.

Diet Study Results

Either variation, a vegetarian diet or a vegetarian diet supplemented with omega-3 oils, works better than the EPA supplement studies where diet wasn't controlled. Inflammation decreases, and pain diminishes; while criteria such as fatigue, morning stiffness, and the need for medication all improve. As expected, a vegetarian diet supplemented with omega-3 oils has a definite edge over a diet that allows poultry and other animal foods and uses omega-3 oil supplements as the single most important factor.

Along with these obvious changes, scientists found that the blood antibodies associated with arthritis (described in chapter 1) fell remarkably. In contrast, non-arthritis-related antibodies remained constant. While this takes us to the very cutting edge of arthritis research, it proves that diet has even more power than expected.

Some of the dietary results derive from the high level of dietary fiber a vegetarian diet provides. Dietary fiber, especially from vegetables, is nature's intestinal cleanser and toner. As a cleanser, think of it as a brush whose gentle bristles have the ability to bind and remove selected waste materials that come from food and are produced in the body as well. As a toner, it binds up to 10 times its own weight in water, which gives the intestine moderate exercise. Oxygen dissolved in the water encourages growth of healthier aerobic intestinal flora. Both these effects explain why the Norwegian research group observed both a change in the intestinal flora and a healthy shift in circulating arthritis antibodies. Their results were one more indicator of a decline in arthritis, and when the vegetarian diet is followed and omega-3 oils are used, the arthritis symptoms decline and disappear completely.

These diet and supplement studies confirm the conclusions from the population studies. Now it's time to consider food sensitivity.

Can Food Increase Arthritis Flare-ups?

Ask an arthritic if certain foods cause flare-ups, and you'll usually get yes for an answer. Ask many doctors the same question, and you'll get mixed messages; some say yes, others say no, and a few admit they don't know.

The Kjeldsen-Kragh research group and others have tested the hypothesis by putting arthritics on an elemental diet, which usually means all nourishment from a liquid. Often the liquid is sent directly to the stomach via a tube, and sometimes it's taken by mouth. Either way, it's not pleasant; but it makes for excellent experiments because it effectively double-blinds a study.

Once a person receives the nutrients required for life, she can consume capsules containing dehydrated food. This rules out taste and other "conscious" factors associated with food. You shouldn't be surprised to learn that food, especially animal food such as beef, causes arthritis to act up. After all, folk wisdom also teaches this concept very clearly. The "test of time" is usually valid.

Other Diet Studies

Other effective dietary studies compared Greenlanders to Danes, Faeroe Islanders to other Scandinavians, and seacoast Japanese to inland Japanese. While members of two groups may be genetically the same, these studies confirm that they do, indeed, follow a diet reflecting their different surroundings. For example, studies on Japanese seacoast dwellers revealed that they eat about three or four times more fish than inland farmers do. In addition, these studies can compare blood levels of omega-3 oils as well as physiological factors.

Comparisons made between people who eat a diet rich in omega-3 oils and those who eat a "Western" diet disclose consistent differences. These studies verified the differences seen in Greenland. In fact, a safe conclusion can be made in several statements that are "practically" true:

- A diet that favors the omega-3 oils reduces the likelihood of developing arthritis in the first place.
- A diet that emphasizes fish, the omega-3 oils, and sensible omega-3 oil supplements, while reducing omega-6 oils, will improve all arthritis criteria, including inflammation, pain, medication use, physical capacity, and general fatigue.
- A diet that emphasizes vegetarian food selections, and is supplemented with the omega-3 oils, will reduce arthritis inflammation and the need for medication, and it will improve arthritis.
- By identifying and eliminating foods that aggravate arthritis, an arthritic can improve his/her quality of life.

Should You Expect Your Doctor to Counsel You on Diet?

Your doctor should always advise you that diet can make a positive difference in any illness. If your doctor says the opposite, please give him or her this book to read. Intuitively, you (and especially your doctor) should know that all your body's metabolic processes are influenced by your food.

Nonetheless, other than encouraging you to follow a good

diet plan, there's very little your doctor can actually do. A modest supermarket has at least fifteen thousand ever-changing food choices. In addition, each ethnic background has its own tastes and desires. For example, how could my doctor, who is Chinese, tell me, an Italian, what foods to select? Worse, some people will eat salmon, others like haddock, and still others are vegetarian. If that's not complicated enough, suppose you're sensitive to fish—then you've got only the vegan or vegetarian route, and how can your doctor advise in that program?

Ask yourself, "How can a doctor specialize in areas as complex as rheumatology or internal medicine and also be a dietitian, nutritionist, and food counselor?" In addition, he or she must prescribe drugs, perform or assist in surgery, and still keep up with what's going on in his profession. Then, when all is said and done, you and your doctor are lucky to get about 15 minutes of discussion time together. About five of those fifteen minutes may be spent counseling. Could even the most gifted teacher impart the information in just this chapter in five minutes?

Only you control what you eat. You can't turn that over to anyone else, including your doctor!

The Bottom Line: Diet Works

This chapter has only one message: Diet works for arthritis. An old saying teaches this: Nutrition is preventive medicine; food and food supplements are the vehicles of its practice.

SUGGESTIONS FOR ADDITIONAL READING AND REFERENCES FOR HEALTH-CARE PROFESSIONALS

Double-blind Clinical Studies

Belch, J. J. F., et al. Effects of altering dietary essential fatty acids on requirements for non-steroidal anti inflammatory drugs in patients with rheumatoid arthritis; a double-blind placebo controlled study. 1988. *Annals of Rheumatic Diseases* 47: 96–104.

Cleland, L. G., et al. Clinical and biochemical effects of dietary fish oil supplementations in rheumatoid arthritis. 1988. *Journal of Rheumatology* 15: 1471–75.

Geusens, P., et al. Long-term effect of omega-3 fatty acid supplementation in active rheumatoid arthritis: a 12-month, double-blind, controlled study. 1994. *Arthritis and Rheumatology* 37: 824–29.

Kjeldsen-Kragh, J., et al. Dietary omega-3 fatty acid supplementation and Naproxen treatment in patients with rheumatoid arthritis. 1992. *Journal of Rheumatology* 19: 1531–36.

Kremer, J. M., et al. Effects of manipulation of dietary fatty acids on clinical manifestations of rheumatoid arthritis. 1985. *Lancet* (i): 184–87.

Kremer, J. M., et al. Fish-oil fatty acid supplementation in active rheumatoid arthritis. 1987. *Annals of Internal Medicine* 106: 497–503.

Kremer, J. M., et al. Dietary fish oil and olive oil supplementation in patients with rheumatoid arthritis. 1990. *Arthritis and Rheumatology* 33: 810–20.

Kremer, J. M., et al. Effects of high-dose fish oil on rheumatoid arthritis after stopping nonsteroidal antiinflammatory drugs, clinical and immune correlates. 1995. *Arthritis and Rheumatology* 38: 1107–14.

Kremer, J. M. Effects of modulation of inflammatory and immune parameters in patients with rheumatic and inflammatory disease receiving dietary supplementation of n-3 and n-6 fatty acids. 1996. *Lipids* 31: Suppl. S, 243–47.

Lau, C. S., et al. Effects of fish oil supplementation on nonsteroidal antiinflammatory drug requirement in patients with mild rheumatoid arthritis: a double-blind placebo controlled study. 1993. *British Journal of Rheumatology* 32: 982–89.

Lau, C. S., M. McLaren, and J. J. Belch. Effects of fish oil on plasma fibrinolysis in patients with mild rheumatoid arthritis. 1995. *Clinical and Experimental Rheumatology* 13: 87–90.

Magaro, M., et al. Influence of diet with different lipid composition on neutrophil chemiluminescence and disease activity in patients with rheumatoid arthritis. 1988. *Annals of Rheumatoid Diseases* 47: 793–96.

Nielsen, G. L., et al. The effects of dietary supplementation with n-3 polyunsaturated fatty acids in patients with rheumatoid arthritis: a randomized, double-blind trial. 1992. *European Journal of Clinical Investigations* 22: 687–91.

Sköldstam, L., et al. Effect of six months of fish oil supplementation in stable rheumatoid arthritis. A double-blind, controlled study. 1992. *Scandinavian Journal of Rheumatology* 21: 178–85.

Uhlig, T. Omega-3 fatty acids (fish oil) in the clinical use. 1995. *Deutsch Medical Wochenschrift* 120: 1262–63.

van der Temple, H., et al. Effects of fish oil supplementation in rheumatoid arthritis. 1990. *Annals of Rheumatoid Diseases* 49: 76–80.

Diet Studies

Haugen, M. A. A pilot study of the effect of an elemental diet in the management of rheumatoid arthritis. 1994. *Clinical and Experimental Rheumatology* 12: 275–79.

Haugen, H. A., et al. Changes in plasma phosphilip fatty acids and their relationship to disease activity in rheumatoid arthritis patients treated with a vegetarian diet. 1994. *British Journal of Nutrition* 72: 555–66.

Kjeldsen-Kragh, J., et al. Controlled trial of fasting and one-year vegetarian diet in rheumatoid arthritis. 1992. *Journal of the American Medical Association* 267: 646–53.

Kjeldsen-Kragh, J., et al. Decrease in anti-proteus mirabilis but not anti-escherichia coli antibody levels in rheumatoid arthritis patients treated with fasting and a one-year vegetarian diet. 1995. *Annals of Rheumatoid Diseases* 54: 221–24.

Kjeldsen-Kragh, J., et al. Vegetarian diet for patients with rheumatoid arthritis: can the clinical effects be explained by the psychological characteristics of the patients? 1994. *British Journal of Rheumatology* 33: 569–75.

Kjeldsen-Kragh, J., et al. Changes in laboratory variables in rheumatoid arthritis patients during a trial of fasting and one-year vegetarian diet. 1995. *Scandinavian Journal of Rheumatology* 24: 85–93.

Peltonen, R., et al. Changes of facial flora in rheumatoid arthritis during fasting and a one-year vegetarian diet. 1994. *British Journal of Rheumatology* 33: 683–743.

Can Food Cause Flare-ups?

Stephenson, Joan. Fishing for a dietary connection? Arthritis and diet. 1993. *Harvard Health Letter,* 18, no. 9: 4–5.

7

Why Diet? Why Not Just Take Omega-3 Oil Supplements?

Clinical studies that focus on omega-3 oil supplements make a diet plan look difficult, if not complex. The experiences seen in Greenland, Japan, and the Faeroe Islands, and other comparative studies, proved an important point: If you make a complete dietary and supplement commitment, you will get better results than by simply cutting out meat and using omega-3 oil supplements. By using only supplements, you run a substantial risk of never achieving your maximum potential. In a way, you'd be using a food supplement (omega-3 oils) as if it were a medicine, which it isn't. You've heard this before: "You've got to eat, so do it correctly and maximize your results." I always say: "In nutrition, teamwork is essential, and you should optimize all nutrients to get the best results."

More important, perhaps, diet can accomplish something supplements cannot. Glance again at chapter 5 and recognize that eicosapentaenoic acid (EPA) competes with arachidonic acid (AA) to make either a good or bad prostaglandin. Diet makes that competition work in your favor by minimizing AA and maximizing EPA on a consistent basis. Sensible supplementation with omega-3 oils can make a diet work much better than doing either one alone, but only diet can reduce the level of AA. A dietary approach is "holistic," in that it uses all the research findings and doesn't focus on only one path.

Total Body Fat

Now that you understand the basis of inflammation, you
need to know that there's another approach, along with
changing your diet, that will yield significant benefits—to reduce total body fat to a reasonable level. Even if you're already at your normal body weight and are inactive, you
could still benefit from an exercise plan. For everyone else,
excess weight makes arthritis worse by stressing the weight-
bearing joints, and increasing the likely spread to the other
joints. In addition, extra body fat is an AA reservoir.

The only way to reduce total body fat is by combining diet
and exercise. You don't have to become an athlete; you just
have to do regular, moderate exercise, such as a brisk walk.
Swimming is better yet. And you can develop an excellent
workout with one of the many fat-burning and muscle building devices. Chapter 18 is devoted to exercise and will cover
these options in detail.

Exercise and keeping dietary fat and total calories down—
this combination will help maximize the desired results: freedom from the debilitating effects of arthritis. A secondary
benefit is a reduction in the risk of the "big three"—heart attack, stroke, and cancer—killers that gain strength from excess body fat and are diminished by optimizing body fat.

Dietary Fiber

Typical eating patterns supply less than 50 percent of the
daily dietary fiber an average person requires, let alone someone with arthritis. Many arthritis folk remedies increase dietary fiber, especially a type we call soft or soluble fiber.
Increasing fiber helps explain the excellent results arthritics
get with vegetarian diets. Therefore, by increasing dietary
fiber, you achieve a double-barreled result: a bulkier, lower
calorie diet and some arthritis relief. Although fiber supplements can help a great deal, dietary fiber is best.

A high-fiber diet is low in fat and accelerates the shifting
of fat reserves so that they will contain EPA. Hence, you reduce inflammation by using nutritional teamwork.

In addition, fiber helps remove the body wastes that are

excreted along with bile through the bile duct. These wastes, bound and removed by the correct fiber balance, can aggravate arthritis when they are reabsorbed farther down the intestinal tract and recirculated.

Numerous studies have proven that when six grams of fiber supplements are taken daily, bile wastes are increased so effectively that blood cholesterol drops by about 10 percent. The same and other studies indicate that indirect benefits include less arthritis pain and fewer flare-ups. The improvement in arthritis results from the removal of bile and other wastes from the intestinal tract.

As an interesting aside, these studies have similarly shown a reduction in the risk of cancer (including breast and prostate cancer) and heart disease, and an improvement in skin tone. It all adds up to the need for a high-fiber diet *and* sensible fiber supplements (about six grams daily).

Food Sensitivity

Arthritis flare-ups can be precipitated by a reaction to food, as clinical research proves and most people learn by experience. Some experts designate entire food families off limits for arthritics; but there's not much substance to those notions. Rather, the scientific evidence is that food, especially meat and other animal-based foods, can aggravate arthritis. The ability of food to cause arthritis flare-ups and aggravate arthritis is a vast area of fertile research that remains to be done. When we discover how specific food factors aggravate such a major illness as arthritis, we will know much more about the workings of food sensitivities.

Don't confuse allergy with sensitivity. An allergy causes a significant response. For example, someone allergic to peanuts will swell up, or her eyes will become swollen shut, or she'll break out in hives with even the smallest consumption. At its extreme, an allergy can cause severe shock, and on rare occasions, even death. That's a far cry from eating something today and having an arthritis flare-up in a day or two.

A sensitivity, in contrast, is more subtle. It doesn't act like an allergy but it causes a response. Food sensitivities can be detected by simply keeping a food diary and identifying any that might affect you. For example, when I wrote my first book on arthritis and had people keep a careful food diary, what emerged surprised most of the followers.

Those who had sensitivities learned that there's a threshold. For instance, several people wouldn't respond to one or two eggs, but if they had three or four eggs in a two-day period, the arthritis would flare up. Similarly for some vegetables and fruits.

Lactose intolerance is an excellent example. People sensitive to milk usually can't tolerate the milk sugar, lactose. Symptoms include diarrhea, cramps, and excessive gas. A recent study published in the *New England Journal of Medicine* demonstrated that most lactose-intolerant people can still drink about seven ounces of milk daily without feeling the effects. That translates to being able to use milk on cereal or in coffee, or eating a modest amount of yogurt. With a little simple planning, lactose intolerance can be managed.

So food sensitivities are a dietary issue. You've got to detect them through diet analysis, and you've got to compensate for them in your planning. No amount of supplements will make up for that.

Now we're ready for Part 2 and the diet program.

Inflammation Fighters: Six Ways to Relieve Inflammation and Pain

Start converting what you have learned into action. The "inflammation fighters" explained here are dietary factors you can apply every time you eat a meal, have a snack, or take a food supplement. Like any good habit, they can change your life for the better. You won't notice the benefits immediately, but they will accumulate like a small amount of money added to a savings account each day.

8

Inflammation Fighter #1: Excellent Protein Sources

Stop Red Meat

Ten to 15 percent of the calories in your new diet will come from protein. If you're typical, you will think of meat (i.e., beef—perhaps a nice thick steak—pork, or veal). Perhaps you even think of an omelet. The average person doesn't think of fish right away, even though it's the best source of protein available. Pat's letter illustrates my point:

Dear Dr. Scala,

I received your diet today and it's good news and bad news. The good news is that your scientific review convinces me it will work; the bad news is that meat is out and fish is in. Our freezer has six months of beef and lamb. My husband eats meat twice daily, but my family agreed to make the commitment with me. So I will start cooking for myself, but they will have to start later.

To many people, protein means beef. In fact, each year the average American, and person in other "Western cultures," consumes 360 pounds or red meat, 106 pounds of poultry, 250 pounds of eggs and milk, and only 23 pounds of fish. Pat's letter represents a typical response from a person who never eats fish and eats only a little poultry. If your major source of protein is meat, you must change your habit to improve your health.

Eliminate
Animal Fat

Cutting out red meat pays big dividends because your cancer and heart disease risk will also decline. For example, epidemiologists have proven that colon cancer rates among people who eat red meat five or more times weekly is 3.6 times that of those who eat it once a month or less often. It's 1.5 times higher than those who eat red meat twice weekly. Mortality rates from heart disease are similar in the same comparison. So if your family is like Pat's, everyone will gain by not eating red meat. You can gain even more.

Careful studies have shown that factors in red meat aggravate arthritis in up to 20 percent of sufferers. This means that red meat will probably cause your arthritis to flare up; or if it's "chronic" (always painful), red meat will make it even worse.

Fish Is Best

It won't be as hard as you think. By following my plan, you will gradually change your eating habits so that next year you'll be consuming very little (if any) red meat. Instead you will eat lots of fish, a reasonable amount of poultry, and many more vegetables. Cutting back on milk and eggs (except for skim milk and eggs in cooking) will bring your egg and milk consumption to a reasonable level. You will obtain excellent protein from vegetables, especially beans. Your fish consumption will increase to 150 pounds or more annually! And you will feel great.

We need protein for growth, development, and body renewal; and just about all the foods we eat contain some amounts.

For example, did you know that 35 percent of the calories in mushrooms come from protein? Because there is no fat in mushrooms, the remaining 65 percent of calories come from excellent complex carbohydrates, which include some fiber.

In contrast to mushrooms, ground chuck gets 32 percent

of its calories from protein and 66 percent of its calories from fat—lots of arachidonic acid—and no carbohydrate.

Compare that with a nice piece of salmon. Salmon delivers 67 percent of its calories from protein and 28 percent from fat—with up to 1.5 grams of EPA. Eat salmon just one meal a day, avoid meat and animal products for the other two meals, and you will feel better without doing anything else. If, in addition, you take a capsule or two of EPA and use flax oil, you'll feel *very well*.

> Fish provides the most protein
> for the least number of calories
> and the best fat distribution.

Fish can be classified several ways. The Arthritis Relief Diet tables that follow list the fat, and, most important, EPA content of some commonly consumed fish, all excellent protein sources. This dietary commitment asks you to compare them on the basis of polyunsaturated fat content and EPA content. Tables 8.1 and 8.2 summarize both for you.

TABLE 8.1

Total Polyunsaturated Fat Content of Commonly Available Fish

Fish (3½-ounce serving)	Total Polyunsaturated Fat (grams)
Tuna (canned in water)	3.0–5.0
Herring	2.6–5.0
Mackerel	2.6–5.0
Salmon (canned in water)	2.4–4.0
Rainbow trout	1.4–3.0
Flounder	0.4–1.0
Haddock	0.2–1.0

TABLE 8.2

EPA Content of Commonly Available Fish

Fish (3½-ounce serving)	EPA Content* (grams)
Anchovy	0.7–1.5
Striped bass (fillet)	0.2.–0.8
Cod (fillet)	0.3
Eel (fillet)	0.4–1.0
Flounder (fillet)	0.1–0.8
Herring	1.2–2.7
Halibut (fillet)	0.3
Mackerel	0.7–2.6
Sardines	0.9–1.0
Salmon (fillet)	1.0–2.6
Salmon (canned in water)	1.1–3.2
Salmon, coho	0.2–1.0
Snapper	0.1–0.3
Trout	0.2–1.0
Tuna (canned in water)	0.4–2.6
Whiting	0.9
Crab	0.6
Shrimp	0.5

*Includes EPA and alpha linolenic acid. The amount of EPA varies with the location of the catch, the season, and the food the fish have been eating.

What About Vegetable Protein?

Thanks to modern food technology, you can easily purchase vegetable protein (usually from soy) in supermarkets and from mail-order catalogs, as either preformed burgers or as a dry mix to which you add water to make "meat loaf" or burgers. I take pride in serving these soy burgers and receiving compliments from people who think they just ate a typical hamburger.

Similarly, you can purchase the soy textured as "chicken cubes" or "beef strips." Preparation is simple, and these products can be served in any dish calling for either chicken or beef. Once I served chili made with soy "beef strips" and received compliments on its tenderness. No one realized it wasn't real beef.

The fat content of these products usually comes in at 20 to 25 percent of calories—which is recommended for a healthy heart. Better still, the fat content is mostly unsaturated and contains no arachidonic acid—so it's ideal.

Don't confuse soy protein products with soybean meal, which many people find distasteful and which often causes gas due to indigestible materials. "Soy meal" is ground soybeans, and it contains undesirable factors; for example, it contains poorly digested starches that, in the lower intestine, are digested by the intestinal microorganisms, causing gas and general discomfort. Raw soy meal is not a "friendly food," but when it is refined and the undesirable components are removed, it provides excellent food value.

Alternatively, both beans (with rice) and egg substitutes are also excellent vegetable protein sources. Remember, you only require about 60 grams of protein daily, and the chances are you are getting up to 125 grams, more than twice your need. Some experts also claim that reducing protein is healthy because it reduces the risk of kidney disease. While the scientific jury is still out on that one, the evidence keeps growing.

Protein Recap

The New Arthritis Relief Diet emphasizes low-fat protein. The protein plan is excellent in both quantity and quality. Sources include fish, fowl, and vegetables. Look at it this way: any food that didn't swim or grow from the ground won't be good for you. Limit your use of protein from sources that flew, and be sure to remove all the fat.

9

Inflammation Fighter #2:
Less Fat

Only 20 to 25 percent of your calories should come from fat; on this diet you will minimize animal fat and reduce your polyunsaturated oil intake. Specifically, I want you to reduce arachidonic acid (animal fat) and moderate linoleic acid (found in corn oil and many cooking oils). Remember, they are the primary substances from which the antagonistic prostaglandin PGE-2 is made.

Our objective also bears repeating—to elevate dietary and metabolic eicosapentaenoic acid (EPA) to a level where it effectively competes with arachidonic acid (AA), so that your body makes more of the noninflammatory prostaglandin PGE-3 than the inflammatory PGE-2. Remember, we get EPA from fish and as food supplements; the objective of this plan is to raise EPA in your diet.

A Few Simple Rules

- Get at least three grams of EPA each day in protein-rich fish and in capsules as food supplements; five grams is better.
- Get ALA daily by taking flax oil as a supplement added to foods or in capsules.
- Stop eating red meat and the dark meat of fowl.

- Stop using corn oil in baking. Instead, use olive oil or canola oil, both of which are excellent for this diet, because olive oil is mostly a monounsaturated oil with less linoleic acid, and canola oil contains ALA and not as much linoleic acid.
- Minimize fried foods. If you must fry, try to use a Teflon-coated, nonstick frying pan; and use nonfat frying sprays, such as Pam or an olive oil spray. This avoids the issue of using animal fats or even corn oil for frying.
- Wok cooking is an excellent way to prepare vegetables and fish with very little oil. The best oil for woks is peanut oil, which can be used sparingly.
- Bake, broil, barbecue, boil, poach, or microwave your food—even use a campfire if you can.
- Stop using egg yolks unless your serving provides a fraction of one egg. For example, a cake that uses one or two eggs and serves 10 to 16 pieces is okay. But just eat one piece!
- Stop using whole milk or any milk if it has fat in it. Skim milk and the products of skim milk are okay. Use yogurt or lowfat cottage cheese.

A Milk Tip!

My support for skim milk has almost caused me some blackened eyes, but I've finally discovered the secret of making it palatable. Add nonfat dry milk to skim milk, which will make it thicker and creamier. This combination works well on cereal and in coffee and tea, and it has no fat!

A Lesson in Cooking

Compare a 3½-ounce skinless chicken breast prepared two different ways and judge which is best.

A roasted chicken breast provides 166 calories, of which 126 (or 76 percent) are from protein (32 grams, or half your daily needs). Only 18 percent of these calories come from fat. Even though chicken has no EPA, it's okay for this plan.

As a bonus, its low fat content makes it ideal for eliminating heart disease.

Now purchase the same piece of chicken from a typical fast-food emporium where it is breaded and cooked in fat under pressure. The same 3½ ounces now provides 323 calories, of which 58 percent comes from highly saturated, arachidonic acid–containing fat. Fifteen percent come from the breading, and 27 percent from protein (22 grams).

Worse, sometimes the fat is lard, or simple animal fat, which is a superior arachidonic acid source. Avoid *all* processed chicken and fish for the same reason. No matter what the purveyor says about the fat sources, the fat content is too high. Having spent over 30 years in the food industry, I see their intentions a little better now.

For example, their objective is to make money by gaining market share. This means appealing to "taste" and "mouth feel," which have nothing to do with health. That is why groups such as the Center for Science in the Public Interest show that baked goods are usually laden with fat and that soup mixes are about 20 percent salt (all cleverly hidden by manipulating ingredients lists).

The appeal to taste is a powerful factor in our diet preference. I was once invited to address the Executive Chef's Association annual meeting; I spoke about how they should strive to provide more low-fat and higher-vegetarian-content meals. About six months later, one chef told me he'd been experimenting in his executive restaurant with my suggestions. In his own words, this was the result: "When I served low-fat, highly vegetarian meals, half the food went into the garbage. If instead I served fish in a rich sauce with a vegetable garnish, they licked the plate clean and left their salad. It seems that the more fat I can squeeze into a recipe, the more they like the dish."

His comments describe our tendency to enjoy the wrong tastes. However, we can reprogram our taste buds to enjoy low-fat and healthy foods. It only takes a little time and a commitment to better health.

In both methods of preparing chicken, the chicken starts with less than 200 milligrams of salt. In the first, it stays that way or increases slightly if barbecue sauce is used. The fast-food example finishes with about 2,400 milligrams! Now you know what's in all those secret herbs, spices, and breading that are so tasty. Salt!

Salt is doubly bad. High dietary salt increases your risk of high blood pressure, which is already at risk from the side effects of the drugs you take. Add salt's effect on bone calcium loss, and you increase the osteoporosis risk. We'll discuss both high blood pressure (chapter 20) and osteoporosis (chapters 12 and 18) in detail later, but always strive for a low salt intake.

Bear in mind that a person can get along on very little salt. A teaspoon provides about five grams, which is an incredible excess. Eighty-five percent of all high blood pressure can be controlled completely by diet. However, the diet must get salt down to less than 1,000 milligrams daily and potassium up to at least 3,000 milligrams. If you took a teaspoon of salt on such a diet, you would have no chance of success.

Fish and fowl are excellent sources of protein, with little fat, and they are balanced in sodium and potassium by nature. We can either enhance them by broiling or barbecuing or make them a metabolic nightmare by converting them to high-fat, high-salt foods. Again, food is our personal responsibility.

EPA Supplements

Even if you decide to eat fish often, you will not get the three or more grams of EPA you require daily. The best sources of EPA are oily fishes such as mackerel and anchovies, but most people don't like them. Alternatives such as salmon, tuna, or trout are often unavailable or expensive. Other fish require two or more servings to get one gram of EPA. Like dietary supplements of vitamins and minerals, EPA capsules are actually food in capsule form. Thanks to modern engineering, the capsules are a convenient way to assure you of getting sufficient dietary EPA.

Omega-3 EPA Supplements

3+ grams daily for adults
up to 3 grams daily for children

If you're skeptical about taking EPA supplements, review once more the numerous clinical studies summarized in chapter 6. In all of them, the only effects were positive. There were no negative side effects, which proves they are safe and effective and can provide a higher quality of life. Recognize also that in other studies, related to heart disease, subjects took about 18 or more grams of EPA daily with no negative side effects. Therefore, taking three to five grams of EPA daily is totally safe.

Flax Oil

Adding flax oil to your diet, even if you take EPA, will confer an additional benefit as it helps push your metabolism to produce more PGE-3. Additionally, for those who are strictly vegetarian (vegan), it is completely vegetable oil. Flax oil, which is 52 percent alpha linolenic acid (ALA), is a rich golden color, practically tasteless, and odorless. It can be purchased in liquid form in bottles, so it can easily be added to your food. Don't fry or bake with it, as ALA doesn't tolerate heat well. I personally add two tablespoons of flax oil to my morning bowl of oatmeal or any other cereal. Alternatively, it can be added to salad dressing or used along with vinegar, oil, and spices to make your own vinaigrette. Use it on baked potatoes in place of butter and sour cream. You cannot take too much flax oil, and it will help your program succeed.

Flax oil is also conveniently sold in capsules. Just don't substitute flax oil capsules for EPA completely unless you're a strict vegan. For example, if you take three flax oil capsules or use a tablespoon of liquid flax oil daily, it will count for a one-gram EPA capsule. This three-to-one requirement is because not all ALA is converted to EPA. Even if you use three tablespoons, or 45 grams, of flax oil (equivalent of three EPA capsules), please take one EPA capsule daily as extra insurance. I recommend this because your metabolism might not convert flax oil to EPA as effectively as the average person's, so extra EPA serves as insurance. By the way, reduced heart disease and breast cancer in women are added benefits of using both EPA and flax oil.

> ## Flax Oil
>
> 3 capsules daily
> (equivalent of 1 gram of EPA)

Flax Oil: Marion's Story

Marion is a 50-year-old woman whose arthritis appeared as morning stiffness. She heard me speak and started the plan the very next day. Her results are typical:

> *Dear Dr. Scala:*
>
> *I have followed your program for seven months and the morning stiffness in my hands is completely gone. In fact, I had my rings made larger before I got the plan, and now I have to have them restored to their original size or smaller.*
>
> *However, I use six flax oil capsules daily and one EPA. I haven't had any red meat, very little chicken and mostly fish everyday. So, as you said, there are several ways to accomplish the same results.*

For Vegans—Can I Do It with Flax Oil Alone?

Yes! This question often comes up when I speak on arthritis. Although there are no clinical studies on flax oil similar to those presented on omega-3 oils in chapter 6, reports like Marion's are mounting, as they should. After all, research has proven that our body converts ALA from flax oil into EPA. If you don't use EPA, I recommend three (instead of two) tablespoons of flax oil daily, since no metabolic conversion is 100 percent.

Suppose You Don't Eat Fish

If you think you can't eat fish, don't despair. There are many other foods you can eat. If your dietary EPA is still less than one gram per day, you can simply use EPA and flax oil supplements daily.

However, I must urge you to try fish. It's a rare individual who cannot eat any fish. Learn which fishes agree with you, and resolve to like them. Experiment with different recipes, and you'll probably discover one that suits your taste.

Of all the people who started this plan, none disliked fish as much as Ruth and Fred. Both had emigrated from Germany, and to them food meant meat, and often processed meat, such as sausage. Indeed, they probably ate beef in some form three times daily. An excerpt from Ruth's letter tells it all:

> At first I thought my arthritis and your diet would bring 20 years of marriage to an end. I experimented with fish and vegetarian meals. Fred simply didn't eat them, but one day he tried some "salmon sausages" and admitted they were quite tasty. I noticed he's lost some weight and seems to have more energy. After one year on this program, he only eats meat when we go out for dinner.

Ruth's comments about Fred's energy are not surprising. Saturated fat (from meat) requires more oxygen and reduces the body's energy production; so Fred really did have more energy.

Fat Recap

This diet will provide adequate essential fats and emphasize EPA from fish and supplements. Flax oil is an excellent way to achieve arthritis relief, so take two tablespoons or its equivalent in capsules daily. A major dietary objective is to reduce total fat intake.

Where To Get Flax Oil

Flax oil is probably not available in your supermarket; and not all health food stores and drugstores carry it. An excellent source that is completely reliable is:

Spectrum Naturals   Tel: (707) 778–8900
133 Copeland Street   Fax: (707) 765–1026
Petaluma, CA 94952

They ship via UPS and sell flax oil both as capsules and in sunlight-proof bottles. If you purchase six bottles at a time, as I do, you can freeze five and use one at a time. When you take out the sixth, reorder.

Spectrum is the brand I use. They don't know me, nor do they know I endorse their product. If you know of an equally reliable product, write to me and let me know, so I can tell others.

10

Inflammation Fighter #3: Complex Carbohydrates and Reduced Sugar

The Arthritis Relief Diet derives 60 to 70 percent of calories from complex carbohydrates (which is what everyone should do, even if they don't have arthritis). Complex carbohydrates, in contrast to sugar, a simple carbohydrate, are those that nature provides in grains, cereals, tubers, vegetables, fruits, and leafy vegetables. We also consume complex carbohydrates in some processed foods such as pasta, whole-grain breads, cereals, and baked goods. It's what we do with what nature provides that counts.

Fruit sugar, usually a mixture of intensely sweet fructose and moderately sweet glucose, are exceptions. Fruit sugar acts more like complex carbohydrate in your body because it's enrobed in fruit's special fiber. Fruit fiber is especially rich in pectin, which helps modulate the absorption of sugar; so be sure to eat lots of fresh fruit.

Excess sugar definitely contributes to heart disease, diabetes, and other modern health problems. When not packaged by nature as fruit or other carbohydrate-rich foods (such as high-fiber cereal, high-fiber waffles, pancakes, and so on) sugar gets into our bloodstream too quickly. Excess sugar can cause mood swings, and it definitely induces your body to produce more fat. More fat means more arachidonic acid (AA), and that's not good news for your diet.

Most adults consume 130 pounds of sugar per year; that's

a heaping (to overflowing) six-ounce glass full of sugar each day. Everyone says, "Not me!" In reality, most people eat one-third of it as visible sugar, or about 32 pounds of sugar directly per year; that's only 1.5 ounces each day—say, three teaspoons. Obviously, the rest is in all the processed food we eat. For example, the eight fluid ounces of soft drink we average each day contains almost seven teaspoons of sugar. Bread, desserts, and fast foods contain sugar. It is everywhere, even in salami—which is loaded with arachidonic acid, and is something you should never eat again!

Sugar Substitutes

Although there is not a smidgen of evidence to support the notion that sugar substitutes cause weight loss, they are fine here. Your objective is to reduce visible and hidden sugar. Artificial sweeteners can serve you well if you like to sweeten your food or enjoy soft drinks. Just don't delude yourself into believing you can eat more food as a reward. Rather, see it as a tool to help you reduce your arthritis inflammation.

Blood Sugar and Blood Pressure

Sugar entering the blood too quickly causes a rapid increase in blood sugar. The body responds to this rapid increase by producing insulin, a hormone that facilitates utilization of the sugar. When sugar enters the blood too fast, the insulin response is similarly excessive, and blood sugar rises quickly; then, within a short time, the blood sugar drops below normal, responding to the excess insulin. This produces a condition known as hypoglycemia, or low blood sugar.

Blood sugar influences our moods. After all, it's the only energy source our brain has available; and when it's too low, it's a sort of primitive signal that all is not well. This leads to a number of mood changes, which range from irritability and anxiety to depression. Because 18 percent of people with arthritis also suffer from depression, it's important to monitor your blood sugar level. The rule is simple: Don't use sugar or foods that contain a lot of sugar.

The omega-3 oils, specifically EPA, have a role in depression because they help to elevate brain serotonin. Recent studies have proven that when blood levels of EPA are elevated, mild depression declines. This explains why people who followed the diet claimed they had a better outlook, and why women with premenstrual syndrome feel so much better on this diet. In both cases, the depression either cleared up or became minor. However, don't confuse the mild depression discussed here with severe clinical depression that requires close medical supervision. Severe depression is a very serious illness.

A lesser-known factor is the effect insulin has on your kidneys. The kidneys respond to high insulin levels by raising blood pressure slightly. Though not a problem in most normal weight people, the drugs used to treat arthritis increase the risk of high blood pressure, so it becomes an effect you should avoid. The easiest way is to avoid sugar as one more small step toward living longer and better.

If you are overweight, elevated insulin is more serious because you have a much higher risk of high blood pressure. Getting your weight down is essential, and keeping sugar consumption down is equally important.

Recap Carbohydrates

- On this plan, carbohydrates will account for over 60 percent of your calories.
- Emphasis is placed on the complex, natural carbohydrates found in fruit, vegetables, grains, and pastas.
- The plan helps to maintain constant blood sugar levels.

Inflammation Fighter #4: Dietary Fiber

Our bodies produce many materials that are eliminated in urine, by way of the gallbladder, or through the intestine itself. The important thing is that the system should have available adequate dietary fiber to bind up these materials and flush them from the body. Generally, this means getting 25 to 35 grams of dietary fiber each day from carbohydrate-rich foods and fiber supplements.

The Selective Carrier

Fiber is like a brush with selective bristles that, in addition to moving things along, can selectively bind unwanted materials and remove them from the system. Put another way, there are about five or six types of fiber, all of which have properties we require, and a varied diet provides them all. Sometimes selective supplementation helps.

Hard fiber, the type found in wheat bran, is the "water carrier" that helps to produce regularity. It gives good stool consistency and achieves the objective of regularity. This fiber is found in all plant food, but mostly in the high-fiber cereals, grains, most vegetables, beans, and tubers such as potatoes. You can't eat too much of these foods, and the results will be obvious as you increase them in your diet.

In contrast to the hard fiber, the soluble forms of fiber, such as pectin, gums, saponins, and others, are the best at selective absorption. For example, pectin helps to reduce cholesterol by binding the bile acids produced by our liver from cholesterol and removing them in our stools. Oat bran does it even better, and guar gum even better yet. It also binds the cholesterol and fat that we get in our diet and helps to carry them through the system.

Not surprising, there's evidence that the soluble dietary fiber from fruits and vegetables can help to remove unhelpful by-products of metabolism, which helps arthritics. It appears that some materials, produced by the body and secreted into the intestine by the gallbladder, in the absence of sufficient fiber are reabsorbed and thereby act as antagonists and cause arthritis inflammation. The results of intestinal bypass surgery also reveal that the microflora of the intestine can do the same thing.

In one study researchers used fiber from the desert plant yucca and observed a decrease in arthritis inflammation. But before you rush out and purchase either yucca fiber, alfalfa tablets, or some other mix in a health-food store, remember that you are entering a complete diet plan. Total commitment is your objective, not a quick fix.

Fiber from Food

An easy way to get a good start on the fiber you need is to begin each day with high-fiber cereal. Many excellent cereals are available; Fiber One, All-Bran, Bran Buds, bran flakes, corn bran, oat bran, oatmeal, and barley, to name a few. Add unprocessed bran to pancakes or waffles. Eat fruit on cereal, in pancakes, or plain; eat fruit and more fruit along with vegetables, grains, and tubers at each meal. As your fiber intake improves, you'll become more regular.

High-fiber snacks are excellent all day, but drink lots of water. Water increases the value of fiber. The following list contains some readily available cereals that provide sufficient dietary fiber.

Cold Cereals

Over 12 grams of dietary fiber per serving:

- Kellogg's All-Bran Extra Fiber
- General Mills Fiber One

Nine grams of dietary fiber:

- Kellogg's All-Bran
- Nabisco 100% Bran

Three to five grams of fiber:

- Quaker Corn Bran
- Ralston Bran Chex
- Kellogg's Raisin Bran
- Generic or store brand raisin bran
- Kellogg's Cracklin' Oat Bran
- Kellogg's Bran Flakes
- General Mills Raisin Nut Bran
- Post Fruit 'N Fiber
- Post Bran Flakes
- Post Natural Raisin Bran

Hot Cereals

- Quaker Oats
- Malt-O-Meal Co. Hot Wheat Cereal
- Ralston Cream of Wheat
- Wheatena
- Unprocessed bran
- Miller unprocessed bran
- Quaker unprocessed bran

How Much Fiber? Fiber Supplements?

I'm always asked, "How do I know I'm getting enough fiber?" My answer is: "You should have an easy bowel movement every 24 hours. The stools should be well formed, their color should be light brown, and preferably about 10 percent will float."

Once you're into this dietary plan, if your stools don't fit that profile (except perhaps for the 10 percent floating), start using a good fiber supplement. I don't get overly concerned about the 10 percent of floating stools because it's really "fine tuning" by experts. When you get enough fiber, you will probably notice some stools floating, but if you don't, it's not a problem. Fiber supplements are usually made from psyllium hulls and are often sold as "natural vegetable laxatives" under store brand names. Mix about one or two heaping teaspoonfuls or a full tablespoon with water and drink it about 30 minutes before a meal.

Psyllium provides mucilage, which helps to bulk the stools and maintain regularity. Other fiber snacks, such as fiber wafers and high-fiber crackers and cookies, are also fiber supplements that are simply eaten as food.

An ideal fiber supplement would have the following ingredients: Psyllium husks, apple fiber, acacia gum, guar gum, oat bran, and a few ingredients to help taste and dissolvability. However, it is acceptable to use a fiber supplement that is only psyllium husk. Any supplement should provide from three to four grams of fiber per tablespoon.

Finally, fiber supplements help you feel full and lower your blood cholesterol—two good side benefits.

Fiber

- Double food fiber intake
- Take up to six grams of fiber supplements daily

Water

In nutrition, fiber's teammate is water. Water is another nutrient that rarely, if ever, is taken in excess. Since fiber is the plant material that binds water, it can bind you up if you don't get enough water. In the presence of water, fiber makes your stools soft and consistent; in the absence of water, it can make them dry and hard.

The relationship between water and fiber is made clearer

by this analogy. Milk contains less water than green peas. The reason you don't eat milk with a fork and drink your peas is because peas have fiber, which gives them their shape and holds the water. You want fiber to do exactly that in your digestive system—give stools consistency without excess firmness.

Fiber cannot perform its cleansing action without water; but our requirement for water extends far beyond that. Indeed, next to air itself, it is the most important of all nutrients. In arthritis it is especially important for the elimination of waste materials that, in the opinion of some experts, can cause flare-ups.

Strive for eight glasses of water daily. Although it is best if consumed as pure water, it is okay in the form of other beverages as well.

A Day with 35 Grams of Fiber

Most people have difficulty understanding how 25 to 35 grams of fiber intake daily is achieved, so I've prepared the following table. This "Day of Fiber" exceeds what most people require; for example, a 125-pound woman does fine on 25 to 30 grams daily, while her 200-pound husband needs 35 grams. Therefore, the woman could use this as a guide while cutting back a little here and there, but her husband should stick to the plan.

Also recognize that this is a guide which allows for many substitutions. For instance, beans and rice would be an excellent protein entrée that also provides fiber. That combination could easily substitute for a luncheon sandwich.

You cannot get too much dietary fiber. In the past 30 years, I've never observed a study in which people have gotten too much dietary fiber, and that includes those in which the volunteers took 90 grams daily.

A Day of Fiber

Food Item	Soluble	Insoluble	Total	Calories
Breakfast				
Bran flakes	1.0	4.0	5.0	121
(with ½ cup skim milk)				93
½ grapefruit	0.6	1.1	1.7	39
Snack				
Banana	0.6	1.4	2.0	105
Lunch				
2 slices wheat bread	0.6	2.2	2.8	122
Corn (½ cup)	1.7	2.2	3.9	89
Broccoli	1.6	2.3	3.9	23
Peach (dessert)	0.6	1.0	1.6	37
Snack				
Apple	0.8	2.0	2.8	81
Dinner				
Brussels sprouts	1.6	2.3	3.9	30
Small salad	1.6	2.2	3.8	50
Potato	0.7	1.0	1.7	200
Melon (dessert)	0.4	0.6	1.0	130
Snack				
Pear (crispy)	0.5	2.0	2.5	98
Total	**12.3**	**24.3**	**35.6**	**1218**

Other foods eaten during the day:

	Calories
Yogurt, lowfat	228
Fish	150
Turkey slices	100
Spreads and condiments	100
Total calories	578
Total daily calories	1796

This day is designed to provide enough fiber with flexibility. There's room to have other desserts or accompaniments, such as wine, up to 1,800 calories for women and 2,200 calories for men.

Fiber Recap

- Fiber can help arthritis and contribute to general health.
- Fiber is obtained from cereals, grains, fruits and vegetables. It is also available in supplement form.
- There are many types of fiber and all are important for this diet to be effective. Therefore, I emphasize variety.
- Water is necessary as both a nutrient and teamworker with fiber. Drink lots of water.

12

Inflammation Fighter #5: Nutrient Balance and Sensible Vitamin-Mineral Supplements

In order to function normally, your body requires 19 vitamins and minerals daily in addition to protein, fat, carbohydrates, and fiber. These requirements are expressed in terms of the recommended daily intake (RDI). Vitamins and most minerals are required in very small (trace) quantities. For example, every day you need just 400 micrograms (400 millionths of a gram) of folic acid (a B vitamin). This amount wouldn't cover a dot. In contrast, calcium is required in comparatively large amounts, ranging from 1,000 milligrams (or one gram) for most women up to about 50; after that age it increases to 1,200 milligrams. Magnesium's requirement is somewhat midway, you need 200 to 400 milligrams (fourtenths of a gram) daily. With the exception of calcium (which will be discussed later in detail) and magnesium, all your vitamin and mineral needs can be packed into a single large tablet. I don't believe in leaving anything to chance, so I recommend you insure your diet with supplementation to avoid any possible marginal deficiencies.

Common Questions About Supplement Use

Question: *Aren't excess vitamins and minerals just excreted, making expensive urine?*

Answer: Even if you're starving, your body will lose some vitamins and minerals daily through excretion. Under those conditions, your urine is truly "expensive." If your blood levels of nutrients are high, your urine levels will also be higher; that's normal human physiology.

Question: *What's the upper limit of safety for vitamins and minerals?*

Answer: Up to about ten times the RDI of vitamins and minerals is safe in normal people. Some are safe at many times that level.

Question: *Isn't it expensive to take vitamins and minerals?*

Answer: Our society spends about $1.00 per capita daily on soft drinks. Is that wasteful? The average adult woman spends $1.00 daily on her hair. Is that wasteful? Expensive is only meaningful by comparison. The supplements in this program are less than 50 to 75 cents daily. You've got to ask: "Is my health worth it?"

Nutrition Insurance

"Nutrition insurance" is an overworked slogan, but here it is appropriate. I would like you to supplement your diet with at least 50 percent of the RDI for all 19 vitamins and minerals. Why this amount? The Arthritis Relief Diet will supply the RDI for most of the required nutrients; however, since our major dietary objective is to reduce inflammation, a little variety is lost, and some nutrients—primarily iron, magnesium, and calcium—will fall short. Supplementation is an easy way of insuring that the nutrients are present in adequate supply, and any excess will be additional insurance.

I propose you use a supplement that provides the vitamins and minerals and amounts listed in the following tables. Most supplements will contain within 10 to 20 percent of the values listed here. It is important that your supplement contains all these vitamins and minerals. It is essential that you get them daily.

TABLE **12.1**

Basic Supplement

Nutrient Vitamins	Amount per Tablet*	Percent U.S. RDI
Vitamin A (as beta carotene)	2,500 I.U.** (500 mcg. RE***)	50
Vitamin D	200 I.U. (5 mcg.)	50
Vitamin E	15 I.U. (5 mg. alphatocopherol equivalents)	50
Vitamin C	30 mg.	50
Folic acid	0.2 mg.	50
Thiamin (B1)	0.75 mg.	50
Riboflavin (B2)	0.86 mg.	50
Niacin	10 mg.	50
Vitamin B6	1 mg.	50
Vitamin B12	3 mcg.	50
Biotin	0.15 mg. (150 mcg.)	50
Pantothenic acid	5 mg.	50

Nutrient Minerals		
Calcium	125 mg.	25
Phosphorus	180 mg.	40
Iodine	75 micrograms	50
Iron	9 mg.	50
Magnesium	50 mg.	12.5
Copper	1 mg.	50
Zinc	1 mg.	50
Selenium	50 micrograms	****
Manganese	0.5 mg.	****
Chromium	50 micrograms	****
Molybdenum	30 micrograms	****

* Two tablets provide 100 percent U.S. RDI for all nutrients except calcium, phosphorus, and magnesium, which are explained in the text.
** International Units
*** Microgram retinol equivalents
**** U.S. RDI not established

Few products satisfy the preceding crit
product you select will have less calcium a
this is true, do not worry, because you sho
cium anyway, as I will discuss later. Your di
excess phosphorus and about 20 percent
you need. If the product you select comes to with.
cent of the calcium, magnesium, and phosphorus listed in
table 12.1, it is fine. Don't select a supplement that varies in
these three areas by more than that amount. Products that
meet my criteria are labeled to deliver 100 percent of the
U.S. RDI in a two-tablet serving. Even this won't provide
enough calcium and magnesium, but you can take that as a
separate calcium-magnesium supplement.

Is More Better?

Personally, I take two tablets of the ideal supplement, or 100
percent of the U.S. RDI, daily. I estimate that I get about 70
to 100 percent of the RDI of most vitamins, but not all minerals, from my food. The excess, probably up to 200 percent
of the U.S. RDI or even more, is completely safe; the extra
will do no harm, and there's much evidence that says the excess will do much good.

Most vitamins are safe at ten or more times the RDI, so if
you choose to do as I do and take some extra, you don't have
to worry, as you're not harming yourself. Recent studies of
elderly people indicate that as we get older our needs increase, so taking more than the RDI is undoubtedly good.
The reason we are discovering these needs now is that people are living longer, and early nutrition research was usually
conducted on college-age volunteers.

There's much evidence to suggest that arthritics need more
vitamin E, lots of evidence that we all need up to 500 milligrams
of vitamin C daily, and calcium is definitely a special case.

Calcium

Adult women require 1,000 milligrams of calcium each day
up to about age 50, and then most nutritionists believe that

ium intake should be elevated to 1,200 or 1,500 milli-
rams. Milk, yogurt, and cheese are the most common
sources of calcium; however, a one-cup serving of broccoli
or spinach provides the calcium of half a glass of milk, together with other nutrients. So you should ask yourself if you
consume sufficient dairy products and calcium-rich foods
each day. Common sense says to use calcium supplements
(up to about 1,000 milligrams of calcium daily).

Food Sources for 1,000 Milligrams of Calcium

Food	Amount	Calories	Comments
Cheddar cheese	5 oz.	560	Fat is bad
Lowfat cottage cheese	5.2 oz.	1,066	Too much fat and sodium
Skim milk	27 fl. oz. (3$\frac{1}{3}$ 8-oz. glasses)	290	Good source
Lowfat yogurt	19 oz.	466	Good source

Most government nutrition and food analyses indicate
that calcium is generally short in most people's diets. In fact,
many experts both use and recommend calcium supplements. In addition to the difficulty of obtaining adequate dietary calcium, many lifestyle habits, such as caffeine, excess
sodium, and lack of exercise, cause calcium loss. Therefore,
common sense dictates that one take 400 to 600 milligrams
of calcium daily—as insurance.

Unlike many nutrients, calcium shortfalls are additive.
That means that if you fall short for a year or two, say when
you're a teenager, and then you do it again during your
childbearing years, you will have less dense bones than if you
hadn't fallen short at all. Below-normal bone density is a disease called osteoporosis, which causes much suffering and
even death in old age.

Bone calcium loss is accelerated by caffeine (coffee, tea, soft
drinks), excess meat, salt, and inadequate exercise. However,
much clinical research in many countries has proven that
bone density can be restored by using calcium supplements.

If you drink more than two cups of coffee or its equivalent as tea or soft drinks, take an extra 200 milligrams daily. Exercise is essential in any case.

Magnesium: A Partner with Calcium

Most dietary analyses indicate that we usually fall short in the mineral magnesium, as well as calcium. Since 200 to 400 milligrams of magnesium are required daily, it, like calcium, doesn't fit into a single tablet. Therefore, a good policy is to take a calcium supplement that also contains some magnesium.

Some self-proclaimed experts advise a specific calcium-magncsium ratio for good health. However, a brilliant scientist, Dr. Mildred Seelig, conducted a careful study of adult needs for calcium-magnesium and proved that once you achieve about 400 milligrams of magnesium daily, the body can use calcium very effectively, and there is no need to get more magnesium.

Iron

Iron is another special case. A typical diet contains about six milligrams of iron for each 1,000 calories. Women require 15 milligrams each day. This translates to almost 3,000 calories. The rub is that few women consume more than 2,000 calories each day, hence the shortfall. Even after menopause, when a woman's iron requirement drops to that of men (10 milligrams a day), most don't get enough in food. To add insult to injury, research indicates that some arthritics do not absorb iron as effectively as they should; therefore, making sure you get enough is simply common sense. The multiple vitamin-mineral supplement I have proposed will handle this nicely.

B-Complex Vitamins

Some people feel better if they use the B-complex vitamins as a supplement over and above the basic supplement I recommend. The B vitamins are those listed on the basic supplement as: folic acid, thiamin (B_1), riboflavin (B_2), niacin, vitamin B_6 (sometimes listed as pyridoxal phosphate), vitamin B_{12}, and biotin. If you wish to take more B vitamins, always take them together as a supplement containing all the B vitamins balanced in the same RDI levels, and never more than 400 percent of (or four times) the RDI in a single tablet.

Special Supplements of Single Nutrients

There is a continuing debate surrounding vitamins E and C, beta-carotene, zinc, and a few others.

Vitamin C is one of the most misunderstood vitamins we know. The government recommends 65 milligrams each day, and other expert nutritionists recommend up to a gram. In addition, the medications used in the treatment of arthritis sometimes destroy vitamin C. Therefore, getting enough is an important consideration.

There's a debate between those who advocate up to 10 grams per day and those who advise caution and no more than the U.S. RDI of 65 milligrams. This debate has precipitated much discussion among experts and will probably continue into the next century. The lack of resolution has to do with the criteria on which RDIs are established. Not long ago the deficiency disease of vitamin C was scurvy, but now we are considering other more complicated issues such as its effect in preventing cancer and heart disease.

In the past, it was suggested that vitamin C has some specific relationship to arthritis. We know today that it does not, except that some drugs used to suppress inflammation cause vitamin C loss. The misconception about vitamin C emerged during our study of scurvy. Scurvy's early symptoms include swelling of the joints, especially the knees, which was called arthritis. However, this swelling was the result of a breakdown of tissue from the deficiency; it was not the arthritis we know.

Anyone who uses NSAIDs, including aspirin, regularly requires more vitamin C. These drugs seem to destroy vitamin C in the body, and they increase the dietary need for it.

The Arthritis Relief Diet provides from 100 to 300 milligrams of vitamin C, depending on your use of fruits, vegetables and grains. There is no harm and, in my opinion and that of many experts, probably much good in using an additional vitamin C supplement of up to 1,000 milligrams (taken as two 500-milligram tablets twice daily).

Vitamin E does seem to have an effect on arthritis beyond its importance in general good health. During inflammation, free radical reactions cause damage, and vitamin E can suppress them. A free radical is a compound with an extra electron or proton. It is unstable and reacts readily with other molecules. Free radical reactions are chemical processes that, in arthritis, cause joint damage. They occur in other tissues similarly, causing damage that can lead to cancer. Free radicals are stopped by antioxidants, of which vitamin E is the most ubiquitous.

Careful clinical studies at the Medical College in London, England, established that vitamin E helps prevent joint damage during inflammation. Unfortunately, vitamin E levels in arthritis membranes fall far below normal levels. You don't need a medical degree to conclude that a daily vitamin E supplement makes sense.

In addition, the vitamin E requirement is related to polyunsaturated fat intake, in that research has proven that vitamin E supplements reduce the risk of heart disease.

If you follow this diet plan and use the basic supplement, you should exceed the vitamin E RDI. In my opinion, it makes sense to take more vitamin-E: at least 100 I.U. daily, and 400 I.U. daily would be better. Recent research indicates that people at risk of heart disease can benefit from 800 I.U. of vitamin E daily (a level impossible to get from food).

Selenium is a trace mineral that is generally lacking in people with arthritis because they don't eat sufficient selenium-containing fruits and vegetables.

Folk wisdom teaches that we should eat an apple a day. Although the originator of that advice probably didn't have selenium in mind, it turns out that apples are an excellent source. By eating a variety of fruits, vegetables, and grains, you obtain ample selenium—and, for insurance, use the basic vitamin-mineral supplement described earlier. If you take an additional vitamin E supplement, select one that also contains 25 to 50 micrograms of selenium.

Zinc. Dietary studies have indicated that many arthritis sufferers have inadequate zinc because their diets lack variety— and especially lack shellfish. There is no indication that people with arthritis should self-medicate with zinc tablets, but a multiple vitamin-mineral supplement that provides up to 100 percent of the U.S. RDI for zinc is safe and effective. Zinc taken in five to ten times the RDI amount is in the domain of the physician. This plan and the recommended supplement will provide adequate zinc.

Beta-carotene is the vegetable precursor of vitamin A; consequently, our body converts beta-carotene to vitamin A as it is required for bodily function. Studies of dietary adequacy usually indicate that most people, especially those over 50, get less vitamin A or beta-carotene than they require. This diet should be adequate in beta-carotene, especially if you use the recommended supplement.

Using EPA Supplements

Clinical studies of EPA were reviewed in chapter 6; as I mentioned, I recommend a supplement of three grams daily. However, EPA supplements are relatively new, so they must be consumed with care. Divide 3,000 by the number of milligrams of EPA in each capsule to get the number of capsules necessary to obtain three grams.

For example, suppose your EPA capsules each contain 180 milligrams of EPA; 3,000 divided by 180 yields 17, which is the number of capsules necessary to get 3 grams (3,000 milligrams) of EPA.

Larger capsules often provide more than 180 milligrams of EPA; however, the larger capsule might be difficult to swallow. It is often easier to use many small capsules than a few large ones.

Most EPA is sold as a concentrate from fish oil, which contains DHA as well. DHA (short for docosahexaenoic acid) is also an important nutrient, but it has no known effect on either arthritis or other inflammatory problems. However, DHA does have an important role in the metabolism of EPA.

Don't be confused by the size of the capsule or the percentage concentration. Simply look for the EPA content in milligrams per capsule and take enough to get three grams each day. Taking more than five grams of EPA daily in capsules is both expensive and excessive.

Alfalfa Supplements

When one person tells his doctor, "I feel better when I use alfalfa," it's an isolated experience. When many people relate the same experience, we say it's anecdotal evidence. That means it's obtained not from a well-designed study but from cumulative human experience. Still, such information can often be valuable. First, anecdotal evidence can lead to understanding the role of particular dietary components; second, it can focus attention on serious problems, such as dangerous side effects.

Bill's Story

One day I received a long letter from which I quote a section:

> . . . . *on the other hand, the alfalfa has given me considerable relief with the ordinary type arthritis aches and pain. In fact, if I take fifteen alfalfa tablets per day along with vitamin C and a multiple vitamin-mineral supplement, I get complete relief from all arthritis pain within five days, and I can count on it. Then, I can gradually cut down to eight or even as few as six tablets per day and keep the pain under control unless a bad weather front comes through and the weather changes cause my arthritis to flare up. When that happens, a small amount of aspirin alleviates the pain slightly, but alfalfa relieves it completely within five days when I resume taking it.*

You might think it is in his "head," meaning a placebo effect is involved; except that Bill is a board-certified psychiatrist, and I can assure you he knows better.

People have used alfalfa for thousands of years, beginning with the Egyptians and Arabs. Folklore teaches that it works somewhat like aspirin; but in fact, alfalfa does not inhibit prostaglandin production the way aspirin does.

A research physician from the University of Buffalo Medical School proposed that alfalfa works on arthritis because it contains a bioflavonoid that is chemically similar to an arthritis drug. Though his argument was compelling, I don't believe the large amounts of alfalfa required are consistent with his hypothesis.

Today, people take alfalfa supplements that are made by compressing the dried leaves of mature plants into tablets. And alfalfa, like many other vegetable foods, contains fiber.

I tend to think that the effect observed by the arthritis victim in Buffalo comes from fiber. The idea was first proposed to me by Dr. Hal Ashley, a research physician. Alfalfa fiber is quite unique in its ability to bind bile acids and other materials eliminated through bile. We often fail to remember that the bile duct is an excretory pathway. These bile by-products, called antigens, can cause flare-ups—and even worse, keep the flare-up going. Alfalfa's ability to bind bile wastes has been thoroughly tested, so getting the right fiber should work to reduce flare-ups. In addition, the prodigious amounts of alfalfa used by most people are consistent with this hypothesis. In contrast, if we were observing a drug effect, small quantities of alfalfa should be effective, because if it provided a physiologically active substance it would function like most herbs, which are usually effective at one- or two-gram quantities. Herbal effectiveness is consistent with physiologically active substances; alfalfa, in contrast, functions more like a food substance. Therefore, observations of alfalfa's effectiveness are consistent with the fiber hypothesis.

Dr. Ashley's theory teaches that fiber helps remove materials that induce inflammation from the intestinal tract; but this concept is not new. Hippocrates himself observed that constipation aggravated arthritis. More recently, some physicians have aggressively advocated high-fiber diets for people with arthritis as well. If this theory is correct, the beneficial effect attributed to alfalfa is probably due to the fact that it contains fiber, rather than to any specific, pharmacologically active substance. (I do admit that alfalfa is rich in bioflavonoids, especially the one the doctor proposed.)

Alfalfa fiber is somewhat special in that a large percentage of it is in a group of substances called saponins, which are especially effective in binding bile acids and other bile substances. The only problem with alfalfa is the amount required; it takes 25 to 35 alfalfa tablets daily to obtain sufficient alfalfa fiber. Although this sounds excessive, it isn't, because 30 tablets represents only about 10 grams of dried alfalfa. That's about as much as you'd get if you ate a nice salad of alfalfa leaves as you would a lettuce or spinach salad.

Beans are another excellent source of saponins, which undoubtedly accounts for their excellent cholesterol-lowering properties. So if you don't want to use alfalfa tablets for fear of mooing like a cow, get in the habit of eating beans. Beans come in many varieties, can be prepared in many different ways, and are an excellent source of protein.

Evening Primrose and Black Currant Oil: Gamma Linolenic Acid (GLA)

Another prostaglandin, PGE-1, is derived from linoleic acid (see chapters 4, 5, and 6). This essential, albeit common, polyunsaturated oil we get in many cooking oils and spreads is converted by our body to arachidonic acid (AA). But on its way to becoming AA, another oil, gamma linolenic acid (GLA), is produced. You might want to review this again in the flow chart in chapter 5, but the important point is what happens to GLA; small amounts of it are converted to the lesser-understood prostaglandin PGE-1—which some experts say is antiinflammatory but others say simply modulates the inflammatory effect of prostaglandin PGE-2.

About now you're probably wondering: "What's going on here, and what does this scientific disagreement have to do with me? All I want is arthritis relief." I don't intend to complicate the puzzle; I just want you to have all the information and to be aware that this is an area in which research will continue for many years, if not decades. The bottom line, however, is clear: Prostaglandin PGE-1 does modulate the inflammation caused by PGE-2 when the normal amount is produced. It is also a good idea to take a small amount (one gram) of GLA as evening primrose or black currant oil daily.

Research does suggests this hypothesis is correct and prostaglandin PGE-1 does modulate the inflammatory nature of PGE-2.

As our diet program teaches, if you reduce dietary AA, your body should make sufficient amounts of GLA from dietary linoleic acid. Hence the smallest amount of inflammatory prostaglandin PGE-2 your body makes will be balanced by its noninflammatory counterpart PGE-1. So, if you follow the diet faithfully, don't worry; and you can always take evening primrose or black currant oil for nutrition insurance.

GLA can be purchased as a supplement of black currant (borage) oil or as evening primrose oil. There don't appear to be any safety issues with these either.

> **GLA supplement:**
> evening primrose or borage oil, one gram daily

Additional Supplements?

The practice of food supplementation has grown slowly in the United States, beginning in the late 1920s and 1930s. Now it ranges from the modest multiple vitamin-mineral supplement, which I recommend as a foundation, to all types of single supplements and combinations of various nutrients.

People use other, specific supplements, such as vitamins C and E, because they make them feel better, or as preventives for heart disease and cancer. Give this diet and its recommended supplements a reasonable chance. Extensive clinical research has proven that it takes a good three months to get maximum results. Remember my saying: "Nutrition works in slow motion."

Supplements Recap

The New Arthritis Relief Diet is nutritionally sound, with the exception of moderate shortfalls in iron, calcium, magnesium, and a few vitamins. However, people with arthritis require more of these and other nutrients, and a multiple vitamin-mineral supplement is essential for nutrition insurance.

SUGGESTIONS FOR ADDITIONAL READING AND REFERENCES FOR HEALTH-CARE PROFESSIONALS

Fairburn, K., et al. α-Tocopherol, lipids and lipoproteins in knee-joint synovial fluid and serum from patients with inflammatory joint disease. 1992. *Clinical Science* 83: 657–64.

13

Inflammation Fighter #6: Cooking Oils and Spreads High in Omega-3

Controlling arthritis with diet is really controlling dietary oils. Translate that into selecting the correct fish, EPA, and flax oil supplements, and the correct cooking oils and spreads. It's not as odd as it may sound. For example, you can even purchase high omega-3 cooking oils, mayonnaise, and a spread that tastes like butter.

Following are some recommendations for various types of cooking.

Frying and deep fat cooking: Select oils that work better at high heats. These include peanut, high oleic sunflower, and high oleic safflower oils.

Baking and Sautéing: Select oils that work better at medium heats. These include canola, soy, and walnut oils.

Light Sautéing and Sauces: Select oils that work better at medium heats. These include olive, high oleic sunflower, walnut, soy, and pumpkin seed oils.

Oil for Soups and Salads: When preparing soups and salads use flax oil, canola oil, and olive oil.

Mayonnaise: If you want mayonnaise use low-fat canola oil mayonnaise and canola oil spreads.

Where Do I Get These Oils and Spreads?

You can purchase them at some health food stores rectly from the following company:

Spectrum Naturals
133 Copeland Street
Petaluma, CA 94952

Tel: (707) 778-8900
Fax: (707) 765-1026

Putting Good Intentions into Food

Intentions are terrific, but only actions lead to results. Put your knowledge and inflammation fighters into food every day. But remember one basic principle: Nutrition works in slow motion.

Nutrition is the best "drug" going because it's natural; when correctly applied, its side effects are all good. These good effects, however, build slowly and go unnoticed by the practitioner.

So—you have to have *confidence* that you are building a longer, more abundant life. By doing so, you are gaining freedom from a debilitating illness.

14

Take Control

Food selection is *your* responsibility. An enormous variety of food is available, so if you want to control your arthritis, you must consciously select food and food supplements within the categories I've established in this plan. The objective is to always reduce inflammation to an absolute minimum!

I call foods you should eat the *Do's*. Foods you should never eat I call the *Don'ts*. Similarly, there are some foods you can eat in moderation; these *Caution* foods are for your personal experimentation. In other words, some people can handle them and others will get a negative effect, such as a flare-up. Therefore, keep this in mind when you eat these foods.

Recognize that it is up to you to keep track of what, when, and why you eat; and to make positive adjustments which make you feel better. I can suggest foods and menus, but food choice at any given time is yours alone.

When Should You Start? Intentions Are Good, but Actions Count

Recently I spoke to a women's group in Portland, Oregon, about arthritis, and afterward I attended a buffet luncheon. I got many questions on my way to the dining room; but one woman seemed particularly sincere when she asked, "When should I start the diet?"

I said, "Now! Right now as you go through the buffet line."

About 30 minutes later I saw her walking to her table with enough food on her plate to satisfy a construction worker. What is worse is that she had a huge piece of prime beef, a baked potato with a large dollop of butter, and other delights that made a mockery of her good intentions. I couldn't help asking, "Why did you decide not to start the diet now?"

"Oh, Dr. Scala, I just couldn't resist this prime rib, so I decided to start tonight when I get home."

I would bet that this woman will never get on the program—and ten years from now she will be an arthritic invalid, with a following of family and friends feeling sorry for her.

Start Today

Following this diet plan will put you more in touch with your body and its relationship to food than ever before. I'm sure you want to begin as quickly as possible. Starting a food diary is the best way to jump right in.

A practical way is to purchase a small spiral notebook, preferably about 5″ × 7″, to fit into a pocket, purse, or briefcase. Record *what* you eat and drink, *how much*, *when*, and *why*. In addition, at the beginning of each day, note briefly how you feel—for example, inflammation, morning stiffness in hands, inability to grip something, pain, and so on—and try to compare it with how you felt the previous morning. Do the same thing in the evening, but also evaluate your food in one or two sentences: Was it good for you, was it balanced, did you eat enough, did you eat too much?

Just as each journey—no matter how long—starts with the first step, each life accounts for an enormous amount of food taken one bite at a time. You are now going to make each bite work for you!

How the Diary Works

You'll probably discover that inflammation is brought on by some foods and not by others. Obviously you'll want to eliminate those foods that increase discomfort and increase those that don't. Then you will experience continued results, as food and food supplements make it easier for your body to get the nutrients that have the greatest benefit.

The advantage of keeping a food diary was vividly illustrated when a colleague at Georgetown Medical School and I conducted an experiment with some students who wanted to lose weight. The professor introduced me and told the students I was doing some research on food habits and would like each of them to keep a food diary. Each was given a small diary in which he listed everything he ate or drank, how much, when, and why. Then each night before retiring, each student was required to spend 10 minutes reviewing what foods he'd eaten and write a short 25-word summary critiquing his selections.

Every member of that group lost weight; two years later, all were slender, as the professor who keeps in touch with them told me. They select food better than most dietitians. They enjoy all the food they eat and never went on a diet. Each of them told me that the act of having to think through what he ate forced him to take control. Each recognized what he could do to control his eating habits and still relish food. These new habits now come to them almost instinctively.

Call to Action

I've given you an assignment: Start a food diary. Do it now!

There is no special way to keep a food diary. Just write what, when, why, and how you feel about your food—daily—no matter what you eat.

Get in touch with how you feel.

I don't ask others to do things I don't test myself, so here is a sample entry from my own diary:

Date: May 13

Morning

> *What:* One-half grapefruit, 6 ounces orange juice, oatmeal with zanta currants, 2 tablespoons flax oil, skim milk, two cups of tea with thick skim milk.
> *When:* About 8:00 A.M.—I feel great.
> *Why:* Feeling hungry after writing all morning—starting at 5:30 A.M. Broke at 7:00 A.M. to exercise.
> *What:* Cup of tea, supplements (multiple vitamin-mineral, vitamin C, six EPA, one vitamin E) and an apple.
> *When:* About 10:00 A.M.
> *Why:* As a snack after a phone call from National Nutritional Ed. Soc.

Afternoon

> *What:* Tuna sandwich (with lemon juice, soy oil mayonnaise), apple, a cup of tea with thickened skim milk.
> *When:* About 12:30 P.M.
> *Why:* Hungry. Just finished writing a chapter. Good time to break before going to my boat to varnish the cap rails and to order a new #24 winch for the mast.
> *What:* Tea with thickened skim milk and an apple.
> *When:* 3:45 P.M. with Jim Eddy—just talking.
> *Why:* To take a break and pass the time pleasantly before my search for new winch.

Evening

> *What:* Baked halibut steak (normal serving), salad, string beans, Italian bread, fruit pudding, tea as usual, and a bosc pear.
> *When:* About 7:30 P.M.
> *Why:* Dinner with Nancy and Kim; we planned our Memorial Day cruise from San Francisco to Drakes Bay.
> *Critique:* This was a good day. I feel fine. No aches, no pain.

I know you can do as well or better with your own diary! So go ahead. I have seen people adopt many types of diaries;

some have used commercial daytime planners, others have used elaborate computer recorders. Whatever works is fine. But remember that three things are absolutely essential— honesty, keeping track of everything you eat, and paying attention to the results. Your end-of-the-day critique is the most important step of all. If done correctly, it will give you a better understanding of yourself and your relationship to food.

Since the first *Arthritis Relief Diet*, I've noticed that more diet experts have people keep a food diary. This is a concept that can work for you as you seek to improve a behavioral aspect of your life.

Getting Started:
Checklist

Clean refrigerator/freezer: dispose of or give away all meat, including processed meats such as hot dogs, sausage, luncheon meats, and so on. Keep chicken.

Purchase supplement oils: flax oil and EPA capsules (sometimes sold as omega-3 oil supplements).

Supplements: a balanced multiple vitamin-mineral supplement.

Grocery shopping:
- Fish: especially cold-water, blue-skinned fish, such as salmon, swordfish, and so on. Fresh or frozen fish is fine.
- Vegetables: purchase a wide variety.
- Fruits: same as vegetables; all you want.
- Dairy products: only *nonfat*. Add nonfat dry milk to skim milk for a thicker, richer tasting milk.

Purchase a notebook (5" × 7" is fine) for a food diary!

15

Do's, Don'ts, and Cautions

The following *Do's* and *Don'ts* are your guide to reducing inflammation, so the first *Don't* is *Don't* deviate from the guidelines. The rewards will be great. You will feel the improvement within a few weeks, so start with enthusiasm and vigor.

Do Read Labels as You Shop

There can be eighteen thousand different items in a large supermarket. New selections are added each week, and others disappear. So how can I tell you what to buy? I can show you how to read labels, that's how!

Food labels should provide two very important panels of information—the ingredients list and the nutritional information panel; the format of each is established by the Food and Drug Administration. Therefore, once you catch on, they are all similar.

The ingredients list must contain all ingredients in descending order of content by weight. However, once you get past the third or fourth ingredient, the others are rarely in sufficient quantity to count. Nutritional information panels, which we'll also consider in detail, list calories, protein, fat, carbohydrate, and vitamin-mineral content with reference to the U.S. RDI. Most products now also contain information on sodium and dietary fiber.

Let's look at some food product labels to see how you can use them.

Total Raisin Bran

Nutrition Facts
Serving Size: 1 Cup (55g)
Servings Per Container: About 12

Amount Per Serving	Total Raisin Bran	with ¹/₂ cup skim milk
Calories	180	220
Calories from Fat	10	10
	% Daily Value**	
Total Fat 1g*	2%	2%
Saturated Fat 0g	0%	0%
Cholesterol 0mg	0%	1%
Sodium 240mg	10%	13%
Potassium 270mg	8%	14%
Total Carbohydrate 43g	14%	16%
Dietary Fiber 5g	20%	20%
Sugars 20g		
Other Carbohydrate 18g		
Protein 4g		
Vitamin A	100%	110%
Vitamin C	0%	0%
Calcium	20%	35%
Iron	100%	100%
Vitamin D	10%	25%

Amount Per Serving	Total Raisin Bran	with 1/2 cup skim milk
Vitamin E	100%	100%
Thiamin	100%	100%
Riboflavin	100%	100%
Niacin	100%	100%
Vitamin B6	100%	100%
Folic Acid	100%	100%
Vitamin B12	100%	100%
Pantothenic Acid	100%	100%
Phosphorus	25%	35%
Magnesium	8%	10%
Zinc	100%	100%
Copper	8%	8%

*Amount in cereal. A serving of cereal plus skim milk provides 1g fat, <5mg cholesterol, 300mg sodium, 480mg potassium, 49g carbohydrate (26g sugars) and 8g protein.
**Percent Daily Values are based on a 2,000 calorie diet. Your daily values may be higher or lower depending on your calorie needs:

	Calories	2,000	2,500
Total Fat	Less than	65g	80g
Sat Fat	Less than	20g	25g
Cholesterol	Less than	300mg	300mg
Sodium	Less than	2,400mg	2,400mg
Potassium		3,500mg	3,500mg
Total Carbohydrate		300g	375g
Dietary Fiber		25g	30g

INGREDIENTS: WHEAT BRAN WITH OTHER PARTS OF WHEAT, RAISINS, SUGAR, BROWN SUGAR SYRUP, CORN SYRUP, SALT, ETC.

The label for Total Raisin Bran provides a short lesson.

- Raisin bran is an acceptable cereal for this diet plan. When prepared with skim milk, the fat level (10 calories— just over a gram) is insignificant.
- Fiber delivery of five grams is good.
- Potassium-sodium ratio (1.6) is good.

- The delivery of 100 percent RDA for many vitamins and minerals tells you that it's fortified, but notice that calcium and magnesium—only 35 percent and 10 percent RDI, respectively—are short.

Now on to the ingredients list.

Notice that that first ingredient is wheat bran and other parts of wheat. This is fine, but let's read on:

- Raisins—it is raisin bran, so the fact that raisins are second on the list is consistent.
- Sugar, brown sugar syrup, corn syrup—these are all forms of sugar, and I suspect that the manufacturer selected these sources so "sugar" would not be the first ingredient. In other words, if the manufacturer had simply called all sugar "sugar," it would have appeared first on the ingredient list. Think about this when you read ingredients lists on other foods.
- The rest of the ingredients indicate that there are a host of vitamins and minerals added.
- Freshness preserved with BHT—this means in plain English that butylated hydroxy toluene preserves these ingredients. We'll review these "chemical-sounding names" shortly.

Question: *Would I use Total Raisin Bran?*

Answer: It's a sensible compromise if you like a good tasting, cold, reasonably high-fiber cereal.

Let's look at two other examples.

Kellogg's All-Bran

Nutrition Facts
Serving Size: 1/2 cup (30g/1.1oz.)
Servings Per Container: 17

Amount Per Serving	Cereal	Cereal with 1/2 cup Vitamins A & D Skim Milk
Calories	80	120
Calories from Fat	10	10
	% Daily Value**	
Total Fat 1.0g*	2%	2%
Saturated Fat 0g	0%	0%
Cholesterol 0mg	0%	0%
Sodium 280mg	12%	14%
Potassium 340mg	10%	16%
Total Carbohydrate 22g	7%	9%
Dietary Fiber 10g	40%	40%
Soluble Fiber 1g		
Sugars 5g		
Other Carbohydrate 7g		
Protein 4g		
Vitamin A	15%	20%
Vitamin C	25%	25%
Calcium	10%	25%
Iron	25%	25%
Vitamin D	10%	25%
Thiamin	25%	30%
Riboflavin	25%	35%
Niacin	25%	25%

Amount Per Serving	Cereal	Cereal with 1/2 cup Vitamins A & D Skim Milk
Vitamin B6	25%	25%
Folate	25%	25%
Phosphorus	30%	40%
Magnesium	30%	35%
Zinc	25%	25%
Copper	20%	20%

*Amount in cereal. One half cup skim milk contributes an additional 40 calories, 65mg sodium, 6g total carbohydrate (6g sugars), and 4g protein.
**Percent Daily Values are based on a 2,000 calorie diet. Your daily values may be higher or lower depending on your calorie needs:

	Calories	2,000	2,500
Total Fat	Less than	65g	80g
Sat Fat	Less than	20g	25g
Cholesterol	Less than	300mg	300mg
Sodium	Less than	2,400mg	2,400mg
Potassium		3,500mg	3,500mg
Total Carbohydrate		300g	375g
Dietary Fiber		25g	30g

Calories per gram:
Fat 9 · Carbohydrate 4 · Protein 4

INGREDIENTS: Wheat bran, sugar, corn syrup, malt flavoring salt, etc.

- All-Bran is a very good high-fiber cereal and fine for this plan.
- At 10 grams, the fiber delivery is excellent. At first you might feel full quickly, if you've been eating like average people who only get 13 grams of fiber daily.
- The potassium-sodium ratio of one is acceptable.

Now look at the ingredients list. It tells you that the major ingredient is wheat bran. Since the fiber delivery is 10 grams and the total sugars are 5 grams, the combination of sugar and corn syrup is all right.

A final example is Old-Fashioned Quaker Oats 100% Natural oatmeal.

Old-Fashioned Quaker Oats 100% Natural Oatmeal

Nutrition Facts
Serving Size: 1/2 cup dry (40g)
Servings Per Container: 30

Amount Per Serving	Cereal Alone	with 1/2 cup Vit. A & D Fortified Skim Milk
Calories	150	190
Calories from Fat	25	25
	% Daily Value**	
Total Fat 3g*	5%	5%
Saturated Fat 0.5g	2%	2%
Polyunsaturated Fat 1g		
Monounsaturated Fat 1g		
Cholesterol 0mg	0%	0%
Sodium 0mg	0%	3%
Total		
Carbohydrate 27g	9%	11%
Dietary Fiber 4g	15%	15%
Soluble Fiber 2g		
Insoluble Fiber 2g		
Sugars 1g		
Protein 5g		
Vitamin A	0%	4%
Vitamin C	0%	2%
Calcium	0%	15%
Iron	10%	10%

*Amount in cereal. One half cup skim milk contributes an additional 40 calories, 65mg sodium, 6g Total Carbohydrates, 6g Sugars, and 4g Protein.
**Percent Daily Values are based on a 2,000 calorie diet. Your daily values may be higher or lower depending on your calorie needs:

	Calories	2,000	2,500
Total Fat	Less than	65g	80g
Sat Fat	Less than	20g	25g
Cholesterol	Less than	300mg	300mg
Sodium	Less than	2,400mg	2,400mg
Total Carbohydrate		300g	375g
Dietary Fiber		25g	30g

Calories per gram:
Fat 9 · Carbohydrate 4 · Protein 4

INGREDIENTS: Rolled oats.

This is an excellent cereal. It is simply processed oats and delivers four grams of fiber split equally between the two types of fiber. Although there is some fat—three grams of vegetable fat—it is not a significant amount.

For breakfast, I usually choose oatmeal with one or two tablespoons of flax oil added. Not only is it an excellent all-around cereal for the arthritis plan, but also its fiber helps to lower cholesterol.

Spaghetti often contains no formal ingredients list because it is made only from durum wheat, and there is no artificial coloring or salt added. The nutritional label shows that in a serving of two ounces dry weight, you get 210 calories, seven grams of protein, 41 grams (1½ ounces) of carbohydrate, and only one gram of fat (less than 4 percent of calories).

If the sauce is prepared without meat, or if you make a light clam sauce, you will have a meal with good protein delivery that is high in complex carbohydrate and almost devoid of fat. An excellent choice!

Egg Beaters' ingredients list looks complex but is actually very simple; 99 percent of the product is egg white, and the remaining 1 percent is the artificial yolk created from corn oil and vegetable gums, which are a form of fiber and color.

The nutritional label tells you that the product compares very favorably with eggs for nutritional delivery, without the fat content of the egg yolk—especially the cholesterol.

From this brief review you can see that by reading labels

you can select packaged food wisely. In this way, once you become experienced, you can move through a supermarket very quickly.

Food Additives: Chemical-Sounding Names

At the end of most ingredients lists are the additive materials, used in minute amounts. These are things such as erythroborate, EDTA, hydroxybutylated toluene, propionic acid, monosodium glutamate, and many others, including some coloring agents. I cannot say they are unsafe, because if they had been proven seriously unsafe, they would be outlawed. Personally, however, I avoid them.

I avoid them because food safety is not a firm concept. Additives are usually used to preserve freshness, or as flowing agents so the food will pour more easily, or as coloring agents. They are tested on animals and then used at less than 1 percent of the level to which they become toxic to these animals.

What disturbs me about this approach is that it studies one ingredient under ideal conditions in isolation. It doesn't account for real eating habits, or for the fact that people who eat processed foods are likely to get many different types of additives daily. Add artificial sweeteners to the coloring and preservative additives, and you are in untested territory daily.

I practice avoidance, and I hope you will do the same. In my career I have known of additives that were safe until a new, more sensitive test was devised and that now are no longer allowed. I advise you to use caution and eat natural foods. Begin by cleaning out your pantry, refrigerator, and freezer. Pull out those food items that increase your inflammation; box them up as a gift for a nonarthritic household.

Sensible Caution: Nightshade Plants

Folklore teaches that plants of the "nightshade" family can cause arthritis flare-ups. Nightshade plants consist of some important foods, for example, potatoes and herbs, shrubs, and weeds that are characterized by an alternating stem or leaf arrangement. I suspect that after some of the herbs in the family were consumed by arthritis sufferers and they got a flare-up from them, the entire family of nightshade plants became suspect.

The question of relationship between nightshade plants and arthritis is steeped in controversy. Traditionally it's been speculated that something in them induces arthritis flare-ups and pain. Careful studies show it only happens to 5 percent of arthritis sufferers at most. There's probably a food sensitivity involved, which simply affects slightly more people than average. Therefore, I urge you to explore these foods for yourself. Most people who have arthritis are not sensitive to these plants. Give them a serious try because they expand the breadth of your eating horizons and are excellent, nourishing foods.

Testing is easy; simply make a note in your food diary whenever you use one of them and then avoid it for three or four days. If you get a reaction, an inflamed or sore joint—usually within eight hours—you will know to avoid that food. Caution must also guide you to ensure that something else—such as a weather change or some other stress—didn't cause the reaction. Try it one more time.

The nightshade plant foods are as follows:

Tomatoes. Yes, the old standby of so much cooking and so many cuisines.
Potatoes. Most varieties of white potatoes fall into the nightshade family; therefore, each variety should be tested. And be sure to use them with and without skin. Sweet potatoes are not nightshade plants and are an excellent source of both carbohydrate and fiber.
Eggplant. There are many varieties of eggplant. The most common is the purple-skinned eggplant. Test them all.
Peppers. The pepper comes in many varieties, ranging from the mild green variety to the hot reds that burn your mouth. You should test peppers before rejecting any of them.

Most of the rest of the plants in this family are either ornamental or are used as drugs and herbs and are of no concern to us.

Do Eat Lots of Fish

When you become a "fisharian," your life will change for the better. The following list will give you the basic idea of what fish to select for optimal results. Strive for three to five grams of EPA each day by consuming a combination of fish and EPA and flax oil supplements.

For example, one 3.5-ounce serving of white-meat albacore tuna contains 1.7 grams of EPA, almost your whole daily basis requirement in a modest serving. In contrast, canned bluefin tuna contains 0.9 grams in a 3.5-ounce serving, so you would need to eat a little more. Take three EPA capsules and use flax oil as insurance, and you're home free.

The general rule with fish is that some is always better than none. Fish with blue skin is best, and the colder the water it lives in, the better.

When selecting a fish steak (e.g., from tuna, swordfish, or salmon), always have the salesperson cut the steak closest to the head; it's richer in EPA. You're probably wondering why this is so; I don't have a definitive answer, but the tissue in which metabolism is most active—and since EPA is an important vehicle in metabolism—is where you'd find more of it.

EPA* Content of Fish at a Glance

Finfish (Cold-water fish)	Total EPA (grams per 3½-oz. serving)
High-Fat Fish Mackerel Sable fish	0.9 to 2.6 grams
Medium-Fat Fish Salmon Trout Whitefish	0.3 to 2.0 grams
Low-Fat Fish Bass Cod Flounder Sole	0.1 to 1.0 grams

*Total EPA and alpha linolenic acid

Frozen Fish Is Fine

Modern fishing fleets and fish farms have facilities fish whole or immediately after filleting or cut... steaks. Although fish frozen this way doesn't taste quite the same as fresh, it comes very close. In fact, I know avid fishermen who freeze their catch immediately because it has a better texture when cooked. I believe these fresh frozen fish are better than fresh fish, which have been "fresh" for a week or two; so I recommend you use frozen fish, fish fillets, or fish steaks as often as you can. Do not use prepackaged, breaded frozen fish because you are getting extra fat and calories.

Canned Fish: Selection Is the Key

When using canned fish, select fish packed in brine—often called water packed—if possible; if not, drain off the oil. Canned tuna and salmon in particular are very good sources of EPA, and they cost much less than fresh. When using canned fish for sandwiches, don't add egg mayonnaise—use canola oil mayonnaise or a little olive oil, and some lemon juice. Enjoy the taste of the fish.

Other Seafood: Mollusks, Crustaceans, and Cephalopods

Mollusks (oysters, clams, etc.), crustaceans (shrimp, crabs, etc.), and cephalopods (squid, octopus, etc.) contain EPA, but less than fish, so they are not good sources of EPA. You can assume they contain less than $\frac{1}{2}$ gram per $3\frac{1}{2}$-ounce serving. Use supplementary EPA and flax oil to improve their value.

A Word About Cholesterol

Most shellfish contain cholesterol. In fact, most flesh, whether from fish, fowl, or four-legged animals, contains cholesterol. Shellfish, especially mollusks, have the erroneous reputation of being high in cholesterol, but they don't contain as much as people think. In fact, they have no more cholesterol than fish and are, in fact, low-cholesterol foods. The misunderstanding developed because mollusks contain sterols, materials similar to cholesterol, but which actually help reduce cholesterol.

Shrimp, crab, lobster, and other crustaceans, in contrast to mollusks, do contain cholesterol. They don't contain as much as eggs, but they do contain about 150 to 200 milligrams per 3½-ounce serving. It's simply good sense to keep your dietary cholesterol down, so go easy on shellfish.

Cooking the "Do" Fish

Broiling, baking, and poaching are the methods of choice for preparing fish on this plan. If you wish to fry, do so with canola oil.

Breading can be done with whole-grain dried bread crumbs or oatmeal, and this will also increase fiber intake. If breading requires milk, use skim milk; if breading requires eggs, use egg whites or Egg Beaters or another egg substitute, not egg yolks.

A Word About Garlic and Onions

Garlic and onions impart flavor to anything, especially fish, and can make a plain meal an eating adventure. In addition, garlic and onions contain chemical compounds that help this plan produce better results (discussed later in this chapter). Use garlic and onions; they're great for flavor and health!

Watch Out! Do Not Eat Fast-food Fish

Don't eat fish from the various fast-food emporiums. This plan is all about fish as God made them. What God has made, man can put asunder. And man puts fish asunder by deep-fat frying, usually in animal fat. I'm thinking of the square fish in fast-food emporiums or breaded fish fillets sold in groceries. No matter how compelling the name or the decoration; it's not for you! These fish do not contain EPA; they contain too much saturated fat, are rich in arachidonic acid, and are loaded with salt. They will do more harm than good in your quest to conquer inflammation.

Don't ruin good tuna, salmon, trout, or any fish with rich sauces made with mayonnaise or tartar sauce, unless you make them with canola oil mayonnaise. Learn to use lemon juice, garlic and onions, olive oil, and mushrooms.

Processed Fish

A new product we call "re-formed fish" is now available in supermarkets. This technology uses fish scraps and scrap fish. With appropriate processing, the scrap is re-formed to look and taste like much more expensive fish such as king crab, lobster, and shrimp. In general, this ersatz fish is a good low-fat protein source. Presently it contains no EPA, although someday, through food technology, EPA could be added—when it is, it can be part of your plan.

Fish: *Do's* for Arthritis Relief

Finfish
High EPA

Anchovy	Mullet
Dogfish	Sablefish
Eel	Salmon
Herring	Trout
Mackerel	

Moderate EPA

Bluefish	Smelt
Carp	Sturgeon
Catfish	Tuna
Sea trout	Whitefish

Low EPA

Bass	Perch
Cod	Pike

Dolphinfish
Drum
Flounder
Grouper
Hake
Halibut

Plaice
Pompano
Shark
Sheepshead
Sole
Swordfish

Crustaceans and Mollusks
High EPA

Conch

Moderate EPA

Oysters

Low EPA

Crab
Lobster
Shrimp
Abalone
Clam

Mussel
Octopus
Scallop
Squid

Do Include Fowl in Moderation

Chicken, turkey, pheasant, guinea fowl, squab, and other birds are all low in fat and excellent sources of protein. Select only the breast—leave the dark meat and the rest for others—and always remove the skin before cooking.

Waterfowl is mostly dark meat; the breast is definitely acceptable, although it is richer in unsaturated fat than other fowl. Therefore, duck and goose breast are fine. Apply the rule of not eating the skin; if possible, remove it before cooking.

Do use sliced turkey breast for sandwiches. If the turkey breast is wrapped in skin, simply remove it before or after slicing. Make your sandwiches with canola oil mayonnaise and use lots of lettuce, whole-grain bread, and tomatoes (if your diary tells you they are okay).

Frozen chicken or turkey can be used. Simply apply the "breast only" rule with skin removed, and you're home free.

Barbecued chicken is sometimes prepared before your eyes in glass ovens on a rotisserie. It's okay if you first remove the skin and stick to the white breast meat only.

Cooking Turkey and Chicken

Bake, broil, barbecue, or boil chicken and turkey. If you must fry, use the same rules for fish. Use olive oil and bread with skim milk, egg whites, or Egg Beaters after removing the skin.

Chicken and turkey salad can be prepared with canola oil mayonnaise. Alternatively, plain yogurt and creamy Italian salad dressing are excellent alternatives; they impart a taste that will pleasantly surprise you.

Take-out Chicken, Processed Turkey, and Other *Don'ts*

Never eat take-out fried chicken again. Deep-fat frying is a great way to ruin an excellent low-fat, high-quality food.

And *don't* be deceived by turkey and chicken processed into the form of franks, salami, ham, pastrami, and other well-known *don'ts*. These products are made using the organs, skin, and other waste materials left after turkey and chicken are processed. They may be all right for active children, but they are not all right for you. Don't be deceived; simply avoid them.

Don't use a prebasted turkey at Thanksgiving. The very name should tell you how it is made. The manufacturers know that most Americans love fat, so they inject fat right into the turkey breast. A regular un-"butterballed" turkey tastes just as good and costs less for the same amount of turkey.

Poultry: *Do's* for Arthritis Relief

Chicken, including Cornish game hen, fryers, broilers, and
   capons
Chicken roll, light meat only
Canned chicken, light meat only
Duck, breast without skin

Goose, breast without skin
Guinea fowl, breast without skin
Quail, skin removed
Squab, skin removed

Don't Eat Meat

Your objective is to eliminate as much arachidonic acid and saturated fat as possible. In general, this means red meat is out.

Don't eat beef, pork, veal, buffalo, and lamb. In fact, if the animal walked on four legs, it's out.

If something can be worse, it is organ meats, which should not even be considered, let alone cooked. Avoid them at all costs. Organ meats are the most fat-rich parts of the animal. If there was ever an arachidonic acid storehouse, it's the organ meats.

Processed meats are even worse than organ meat. Processed meat contains about 70 percent of its calories as saturated fat—it's loaded with arachidonic acid. Processed meats are made from all the organs and by-products; consequently, that sausage or hot dog contains stomachs, lungs, livers, kidneys, spleen, and anything else I've overlooked. The only thing left behind is the squeal or the moo, and if they could use them they would.

Processed meat means sausage of any type: franks, bologna, liverwurst, salami, and most other sandwich or luncheon meats. It makes no difference whether the package claims it comes from some exotic animal, such as kangaroo or koala, or even turkey or chicken. Leave it alone.

The use of "turkey or chicken" bologna and sausage is generally a deception. Yes, it is made from those birds, but it's made from the waste, which is high in the wrong kind of fat and only marginally better for you than the same thing made from meat.

Wise men say there are two things we should never see being made: laws and sausage. I think I could tolerate laws, but anyone who's ever seen sausage made (including processed meat of all kinds) never eats them again. Let it go at that.

Occasionally, rabbit and venison are acceptable red meats. They are generally very low in fat and contain alpha linolenic acid and some EPA, because they usually are free-range and graze on grasses, even when domesticated. Although rabbit and venison are not regularly eaten in the average household, they are sometimes available in gourmet restaurants and food shops.

What If You're Trapped?

Occasionally you will be trapped. You will find yourself invited to dinner, and lo and behold, a beautiful roast, chicken livers, steak, or pâté is put in front of you. Don't panic!

Pork with the fat trimmed is often, next to chicken, the best white meat available. A pork chop often has a rim of pure fat—never eat that—but the meat itself is lower in fat than beef and, eaten occasionally, will do no harm. Arthur Godfrey had two rules that always worked: Trim off all the fat; then eat only half of what remains. Willpower to trim the fat and reduce the portion will always help. Remember to critique it in your food diary.

Recognize, however, that after you've been following this plan for a while, eating red meat, including trimmed pork, will often cause your arthritis to flare up. That will subside, and you'll do just fine. When it happens, double up on EPA supplements.

Barbara follows this plan with much success and conducts a self-help group. She explained to me just how difficult it can be.

> *My daughter is graduating from high school, and we were invited to a party in honor of the occasion. The hors d'oeuvres were mostly meat or chicken livers wrapped in bacon. I ate them without thinking and paid the price the next day. My knees and hands swelled, and they hurt. I hadn't realized just how effective this diet was for me until I went off it. I sure have learned my lesson.*

This comment illustrates that no matter how well your diet appears to work, the old problem is just waiting to return. Don't let it.

Meat: *Don'ts* for Arthritis Relief

Red meats and organ meats (canned, fresh, or smoked)
Beef
Lamb
Pork
Bacon
Ham
Veal
Poultry dark meat
Organ meats from poultry
Processed luncheon meats such as bologna
Frankfurters and sausages
Sandwich spreads from meat
Poultry franks and sausages such as chicken franks and
  turkey franks
Poultry luncheon meats such as chicken or turkey salami,
  pastrami, etc.

Do Eat Pasta

Pasta is an excellent way of obtaining both protein and complex carbohydrate. Read the ingredients list to be sure that the first ingredients are, for example, wheat, spinach (in spinach pasta), or corn (in corn pasta), and that if eggs appear (preferably they will not), they are far down on the list.

With pasta the sauce is king, and that's where this plan can become complex if you don't exercise common sense. Proceed carefully.

Tomato sauce is the traditional standby for pasta, and tomatoes are in the nightshade class of foods. I recommend experimenting with all vegetables, including tomatoes and tomato sauce, because not everyone is affected by these foods. I have encountered many arthritics who can use tomatoes with no problems whatsoever. On the other hand, I have met a few who cannot, so you must try for yourself.

The best sauce for pasta is a fish, chicken, or clam sauce made with olive oil or canola oil, added flax oil, and absolutely no cream. Sauces generally described as a "light" clam or fish sauce are superb. These sauces work very well with slivers of chicken or turkey, and green vegetables such as broccoli and parsley. And remember—use garlic liberally! Parmesan cheese is desirable for flavor; just use it sparingly.

The following letter, showing the power of a food diary, explains it all.

> *Dear Dr. Scala,*
>
> *Thank you for sending me your arthritis diet material. I immediately started to eliminate the don'ts from my diet and am taking EPA. . . .*
>
> *I found when I was in Florida that I was not able to eat grapefruit, as my knees and elbow became sore. I found last summer when our tomatoes were producing a good crop, I was foolish to eat a lot of them. My joints became very sore and when I stopped eating tomatoes, the pain went away. I have found that since following your diet, my ankles are not puffy at night as they have been for a long time.*

This letter from Mary, who is 70 years old, brings out two points: It is essential to test certain foods, because what is good for one may not be for another. And it states very clearly that you are never too old to improve your life.

Mary's observation that her ankles are not as puffy is consistent with an Air Force doctor who has used a stricter version of this diet. In his words: "I notice within the first week my arthritis complaints disappear and puffiness around the ankles is gone."

Since we seem to have maligned it a bit, I must say a good word for the tomato. Recent research has proven that eating tomatoes regularly does reduce cancer risk, especially bladder cancer. This is probably due to the red carotenoid pigment, lycopene, that they contain. In fact, men who eat a meal with tomato sauce daily have about half the prostate cancer risk of men who eat it occasionally. So if tomato sauce agrees with you, it *is* an excellent choice.

Caution: Pasta Sauce with Meat

Hopefully, you will have determined by your food diary that tomatoes are fine for you. If so, tomato sauce is the choice for pasta. It is low in fat, low in calories, and nourishing. It can be made from plum tomatoes, regular tomatoes, or tomato paste. Tomato sauce is an excellent vehicle for such vegetables as carrot slices, broccoli, parsley, garlic, onions, and mushrooms. Sautéing of these condiment vegetables should be done in olive oil with added garlic. It can also be converted to a red clam sauce by simply adding canned baby clams.

Never use meat sauce, meat balls, sausage, or any animal fat.

Occasionally pasta needs Parmesan cheese. Use it sparingly. It can be stretched with garlic, parsley, oregano, and other spices and condiments.

Do Use Dairy Products with Caution

Dairy products cause flare-ups in some arthritics. I know of one woman who is even affected adversely by yogurt. In my opinion, it is not the fat that is responsible, but some other material—possibly the protein or, in technical terms, a peptide. The terminology doesn't matter unless you're a scientist, but the point is clear: test yourself. Use your food diary to identify dairy products you can use and those you cannot.

Do try nonfat dairy products and dairy products such as cottage cheese and yogurt made from skim or nonfat milk. Milk fat is saturated fat and usually contains arachidonic acid.

Although drinking skim milk with its bluish cast is not appealing to many, it is better than lowfat milk, as the following example provides. (If you add nonfat dry milk to skim milk, it becomes thicker and tastes like whole milk.)

Consider a breakfast of Spoon-Size Shredded Wheat. This cereal provides 110 calories with one gram of fat; that's nine calories from fat. Nonfat milk has almost no fat calories, so ½ cup of nonfat milk used with the cereal contains only 155 calories (45 from milk, 110 from cereal) and one gram or nine calories from fat. That's only 6 percent of calories from fat, an insignificant amount, and the lowest you can get and *still* use milk on your cereal.

Suppose you use lowfat milk. The same cereal—one ounce with ½ cup lowfat milk—provides about 190 calories, but *now* with four grams of fat (one from cereal, three from milk). This means that 36 of the 190 calories, or 19 percent, come from fat. Obviously, this is not the best way to eat your cereal, because our objective is to reduce milk fat to a minimum while keeping the calories from fat to a minimum. However, 19 percent of calories from fat is still a low-fat meal, and most nutritionists would applaud a person who keeps her fat down to 19 percent of calories. However, our arthritis objective is not only low fat, it's to reduce animal fat to an absolute minimum. Therefore, even lowfat milk should give way to skim milk.

This example illustrates that when you reduce the use of fat-containing foods, you help yourself considerably—with very little sacrifice in flavor. For a flavor bonus, include some fruit on the cereal (e.g., 70 to 100 calories from sliced bananas or strawberries), which will add more fiber and flavor and reduce the percentage of calories from fat to 3.5 percent for skim milk and only 12.4 percent for lowfat milk. You can't lose by adding fruit. If you add a tablespoon of flax oil to your cereal, it becomes an antiinflammation powerhouse.

A better cereal would be oatmeal; Old-Fashioned Quaker Oats 100% Natural cereal provides excellent fiber and about the same calories as the Spoon-Size Shredded Wheat, so the same example would apply. In this case, the fruit choice would be raisins added during cooking, topped with sliced bananas when served.

I get many recipes that people devise to help them get around foods they are sensitive to. A number of people who like oatmeal but cannot use even skim milk use apricot nectar in place of milk. My family tried it and found it quite good. Other people use the nondairy creamers that are available. Add flax oil to these, and you won't know the difference—except for the better health it provides.

Cottage cheese with one percent fat is acceptable if you absolutely need cheese. Occasionally lowfat mozzarella is acceptable, but it should be used sparingly. All other cheeses, except ricotta, and Parmesan sparingly on pasta, are *Don'ts* on this diet.

Ricotta cheese, if used in a meal such as stuffed shells or stuffed manicotti, is okay if the meal also contains generous servings of vegetables; and if the pasta portion is small.

Ricotta can be mixed with cottage cheese, parsley, and broccoli (and, of all things, unprocessed bran), and carbohydrate calories can be added by an appropriate tomato sauce. Careful planning is required to reduce the calories from fat to an absolute minimum—strive for no more than 15 percent of the total.

High Fat: A Dairy Wasteland

Don't eat high-fat dairy products. Once you get past the non-fat dairy products made with skim milk (such as cottage cheese or yogurt), dairy becomes a wasteland of *Don'ts* that include ice cream, cheese, and most other dairy products.

Some of the most popular dairy foods are desserts such as ice cream. Dairy fat, as you know, should be avoided; therefore, most of these desserts are not acceptable. A good alternative is sherbet, which can be used as often as you wish. All flavors are fine, and they are especially nutritious when topped with fruit.

Pudding made with skim milk is another acceptable dessert. Let's do some arithmetic: ½ cup butterscotch pudding made from a mix with lowfat milk contains 4.7 grams of fat; that's 42 calories from fat out of a total of 171 calories (most from carbohydrate), or only 25 percent of calories from fat. Add some fruit, such as bananas, and you've reduced the fat to less than 20 percent of calories. Use skim milk, and the pudding is great!

Yogurt from skim milk or nonfat dry milk is an excellent choice. It is especially good if fruit is included. However, yogurt made from whole milk should not be used.

If you look through various cookbooks you'll find all kinds of dessert recipes that make use of skim milk and cottage and ricotta cheese and are low in fat. Just remember to keep the fat calories as low as possible and always less than 25 percent of the total calories. By topping with fruit, you introduce more carbohydrate, reducing the fat-to-calorie percentage, and dietary fiber.

Special Treats

Occasionally have ice milk for dessert and top with fruit; it may lift your spirits.

And *occasionally* you can eat a vegetarian pizza with skim milk mozzarella cheese, lots of garlic, onions, green peppers, and olives. Cook it on a "pizza brick" to help reduce the oil content of the final dish.

Don't Use Whole Eggs

Egg white is fine whenever eggs are required (e.g., recipes, breading mix, etc.). The egg yolk is the problem; so don't eat it except occasionally.

Do use egg substitutes whenever possible. Products such as Egg Beaters are excellent for recipes that use the whole egg (scrambled eggs, omelets, and French toast).

Dairy Product *Do's* for Arthritis Relief

Cheese

Cottage cheese (lowfat or skim milk)   Parmesan (grated)—sparingly
Mozzarella (skim milk)—limited intake   Ricotta (skim milk)

Milk

Skim   Skim made from dry milk
Skim protein fortified

Yogurt

Skim milk yogurt

Dairy Desserts

Ice milk—occasionally
Sherbet

Dairy Product *Don'ts* for Arthritis Relief

Whole milk   Goat milk
Lowfat (2% fat) milk   Yogurt from whole milk

Homogenized milk
Evaporated and condensed milk
Buttermilk
Butter

Cheese from whole milk
Egg yolks

Check Your Food Diary

Occasionally use egg yolks in recipes in which there are at least four servings for every egg yolk. Better yet, *don't* use whole eggs for cooking unless the yolk is absolutely necessary, and the final product (e.g., a cake) will be divided into many pieces—in that case, you're actually eating about one-tenth of an egg.

Some "dietary experimentalists" tell me they can eat an egg occasionally. But they keep watch in the food diary, and if they don't put at least one day between the eggs, they see swelling and flare-up. Trial and error is the key to success.

Do Use Vegetable Protein Substitutes

Soy protein products made to meet vegetarian needs are excellent on this diet plan. They are available in most supermarkets and by catalog. An excellent source is:

Harvest Direct
P.O. Box 4514
Decatur, IL 62525-4514

Tel: 1-800-835-2867

Textured vegetable protein is the correct name for these products, which are usually made from purified soy protein. The protein is excellent in quality and low in fat and contains no arachidonic acid. It comes in several forms:

- *Burger/meat loaf mix,* when mixed in water, makes the equivalent of ground beef, which can be used to make hamburgers or a meatloaf. It comes in a variety of flavors: plain, Italian, or with herbs and spices. A seasoning mix can be purchased that even imparts the flavor of real breakfast sausage. I've served it often, and no one knew the difference.

- *"Chicken" chunks* are mixed with a small amount of water (a tablespoon of vinegar helps) to make chunks of excellent imitation white meat chicken. This can be cooked and used in recipes whenever chicken is called for. Soy chicken chunks require a little experimentation to get everything just right.

- *"Beef" strips* are hydrated in water and can be used whenever a recipe requires beef. In general, they can be cooked in stew, stroganoff, and chili, or after cooling used in salad or as slices on a sandwich.

You can serve any of these products to guests, and they will compliment you on the excellent burger, beef or chicken. When told the actual ingredient, they usually ask where you bought the products so they can purchase them.

No, I am not advertising—nor do I get these products free. In fact, the manufacturer doesn't know me at all. I simply use these products because they work and are excellent sources of low-fat protein.

Do Eat Generous Amounts of Cereals and Grains

Do eat lots of cereals and grains. You can't use too much, no matter how hard you try. Occasionally people are sensitive, even allergic, to such foods. If you suspect sensitivity, use your food diary to identify the culprits.

Breakfast cereals are excellent, especially those made from whole grains. The objective of eating cereals is to obtain dietary fiber, especially soluble dietary fiber (such as gums), which is found in oatmeal. Learn what to look for on the cereal's ingredients list.

The first ingredient should be the substance of the cereal; for example, oats, corn bran, wheat.

Preferably the cereal will contain neither sugar nor corn syrup, but if it does contain one of these (not both), it is still okay, because getting enough fiber is the important objective.

There should be a listing that shows the amount of dietary fiber per serving. On the Arthritis Relief Diet you should select cereals that provide at least four grams of fiber and preferably more—up to nine grams.

Eat breakfast cereals with skim milk and fruit, and use sugar sparingly; try brown sugar, honey, or maple syrup instead of granulated sugar.

Most Americans think of cereals and grains only as something to eat for breakfast. But these excellent sources of fiber, complex carbohydrate, and protein also include the following foods good for any mealtime:

Barley, especially pearled barley.

Corn, from corn on the cob to cornmeal. Corn pasta is available for those who have severe allergies to wheat. It requires special cooking but is a fine way to add more vegetables to your diet.

Rice, rich in carbohydrate and fiber; and, with appropriate accompaniments, protein. Rice has everything going for it and nothing against it. It comes in many forms, including long-grain, brown, wild, and polished.

Wheat, or wheat germ, in the form of cooked cracked wheat (use as a side dish like rice or potatoes). Add a sauce that is low in fat or mix the wheat with rice.

Whole-grain Bread, delicious with spreads such as olive oil, peanut, or sesame oil. Unsalted peanut butter or almond butter are also acceptable.

Don't Go Wrong

Don't use homogenized or whole milk on breakfast cereals. Learn to do without sugar.

Occasionally take a break from the standard. Remember that this is a lifelong commitment; therefore, try different foods such as grits, barley, and so on. Switch around and let variety work for you. Cereals and grains can only help and never hurt in your search for relief, so use them generously.

Grain and Grain Products: *Do's* for Arthritis Relief

Breads and Rolls

Bagel
Biscuits (nonbuttermilk)
Brown bread
Brown bread with raisins
Cracked wheat
French
Fresh Horizons white or wheat
Hollywood dark and light
Honey wheatberry

Italian
Matzo
Mixed grain
Raisin
Rye (all types)
Sourdough
Wheat
Wheatberry
White (low sodium)

Crackers

Melba toast
Rice wafer
Rusk

RyeKrisp
Triscuits
Zwieback

Dinner Rolls

Brown and serve
French
Raisin
Rye, hard

Wheat
White, hard
Whole wheat

Muffins

English muffins (plain and sourdough)
Bran

Whole wheat

Noodles

Asian dry
Rice
Saimin

Soba
Enriched egg

Pancakes

Most pancakes are made from mixes. Unprocessed bran can be added to the batter to increase their dietary fiber. Egg Beaters can replace eggs in the mix.

Plain
Buttermilk
Buckwheat

Cornmeal
Soy

Grain and Grain Products: *Do's* for Arthritis Relief

Waffles

Waffles are generally higher in fat than pancakes. Unprocessed bran can be added to the batter; Egg Beaters can replace eggs.

Cooked Cereals

Barley	Oatmeal
Buckwheat	Ralston
Cream of wheat	Whole wheat

Cold (Ready to Eat) Cereals

All-Bran (all brands including extra fiber)	Oat bran
40% Bran flakes (all brands)	Wheaties
Bran Buds	Most
Raisin bran	Nutri-grain wheat and raisins
Shredded wheat	
Corn Bran	

Do Include Lots of Vegetables

If I have things my way, you will learn that with the exception of breakfast, you should eat a vegetable or two with each meal, together with a green salad. And breakfast should always include fruit. The rewards are more than worth the effort and investment.

There is no end to the variety of vegetables in this world, and no end to their varied colors and tastes. They all provide various levels of dietary fiber and are generally good sources of potassium, the B vitamins, and vitamin C. *Don't* forget, though, that the nightshade vegetables present a problem to some people.

The best way to prepare vegetables is to steam them lightly so they are still crunchy. Stir-frying is excellent, but only if you use canola or Puritan oil. Soybean or peanut oil are okay, but they are second best, and corn oil is out. Before serving, stir in some flax oil.

Frozen vegetables are fine. They retain their nutrients, fiber, and taste, contrary to popular opinion—or should I say misconception. They offer more nutrients than their "fresh" counterparts (because they are usually flash-frozen after being picked, while fresh can sometimes be sitting around in transport, etc., before reaching the market), even if they have been sitting in a frozen food compartment in a supermarket or on a refrigerated truck for a few days or even weeks.

Canned vegetables are not as good as frozen because they usually contain salt and sometimes sugar. Nevertheless, canned vegetables contain about as much fiber as their frozen or fresh counterparts. If there are no alternatives, then use them.

Beans

Do remember that beans deserve a special place in your diet. A serving of kidney beans with 120 calories provides about 25 percent as protein, 85 percent as carbohydrate, and no fat. Each 3½-ounce serving provides five grams of dietary fiber. Therefore, a meal of beans, rice, a salad, and another vegetable is, by any standards, excellent.

Salad possibilities with beans are also appealing—use olive, canola, or Puritan oil in the dressing, and add some flax oil.

For years people have called beans the musical fruit. This is a polite reference to the flatulence, the gas that develops when people eat beans for a meal. Beans contain carbohydrates that cause flatulence; but when the microflora of the intestines acclimate to them, the flatulence disappears.

Canned beans are fine; just select ones that contain no pork or other animal products. When fat is added, it destroys the quality of this great food. Baked beans made with molasses or other non–animal fat components are excellent.

Garlic, Onions, Chives, Shallots, and So On

Do use garlic and onions.

Perhaps only people in Gilroy, California, the "garlic capital," sit down to fried garlic and sautéed onions, but if more people did, they would be doing themselves a favor. These two foods contain materials that help the prostaglandins perform their functions.

In fact, research has shown that natural materials in garlic and onions can actually act, to some extent, as prostaglandins. You simply can't use too much garlic, onions, and other condiments such as shallots and leeks. You must, however, take into account your friends, next of kin, loved ones, business associates, and anyone else who might come in contact with your breath and body odor.

Garlic Magic

Since 1650 B.C. in Egypt, garlic has been credited with unique health properties. These properties helped Roman legions win wars by keeping soldiers healthy and able to fight. In World War I, garlic oil was a field surgeon's main defense against wound infection, since it contains natural antibiotics. During the great plagues, garlic was mixed in wine as an elixir and saved many lives by preventing infection. Garlic has stood the tests of time and modern research.

Careful research has proven that common cold and flu viruses are stopped by garlic; similarly, for the most common yeast infection, Candida albicans. Hence, folk wisdom about the preventive properties of garlic is correct.

Most recently, scientists have proven that garlic's unique antioxidants help prevent cancer and slow tumor growth, confirming observations first made by early Egyptian physicians. The same qualities in garlic help reduce blood pressure and lower cholesterol. Therefore, garlic also helps prevent heart disease.

Knowledge about garlic handed down through the ages has stood the tests of both the "school of hard knocks" and rigorous research by modern scientists. Indeed, garlic seems even more magical than folk wisdom teaches.

How Much Garlic Can You Eat?

A careful review of the research suggests that one larg of garlic daily is simply a good, common-sense health hab with lots of benefits. But garlic's active materials have a powerful odor, and that's where the garlic magic runs head long into modern life. Who eats a raw clove daily? Who wants to? Who wants you around if you do?

Garlic supplements are the modern equivalent of a very generous garlic clove. The odor is usually enrobed in a natural coating, so it's released in the body where it does its job, and no one can tell you've had garlic. A tablet a day will provide many benefits; and while protecting your health, you won't offend anyone. Still, the most enjoyable way to eat garlic is to use it generously in cooking.

Important Reminders on Cooking Vegetables

Cooking vegetables is just about as simple or as elaborate as you want it to be. Steam until crisp, but cooked; boil if you must, or stir-fry in olive, canola or Puritan oil; add garlic to taste.

Don't cook vegetables in corn oil, butter, animal fat, or other fatty materials. Olive, canola, or Puritan oil are the choices for cooking oil.

Occasionally try something really new. There is such a variety of vegetables available; take time to test all of them. You can't exhaust the variety in a lifetime: jicama, Jerusalem artichoke, water chestnuts, and salsify, to name but a few.

Vegetables: *Do's* for Arthritis Relief

Alfalfa sprouts
Artichokes
Asparagus
Avocado
Bamboo shoots
Beans (canned with molasses or brown sugar)
Beans, white cooked
Beets
Beet greens

Black-eyed peas
Broccoli
Brussels sprouts
Butter beans
Cabbage
Carrots
Cauliflower
Celeriac root
Celery

Chard
Chicory
Chives
Collard greens
Corn, white or yellow
Cowpeas
Cucumber
Dandelion greens
Eggplants
Endive
Fennel
Garbanzo beans (chickpeas)
Ginger root
Green beans (Italian and snap)
Hominy
Jerusalem artichoke
Kale
Kidney beans, red
Kohlrabi
Leeks
Lentils
Lettuce
Lima beans
Mung bean sprouts
Mushrooms
Mustard greens
Mustard spinach
Okra

Onions
Parsley
Peas
Pepper, bell
Pimientos
Potato, white (caution)
Pumpkin
Purslane
Radishes, red
Rhubarb
Scallions
Shallots
Snow peas
Spinach
Squash (acorn,
    butternut, hubbard,
    zucchini, summer,
    and winter)
Sweet potato
Turnip greens
Water chestnuts
Watercress
Wax beans
Winged beans
Yams
Yambeans
Yautia

Do Add Fruit

Do become passionate about fruit. You can never eat too much fruit! The variety is enormous, and it's all great for you. Fruit, for all practical purposes, has no fat, and is high in soluble fiber, which is excellent for arthritis—and the fiber moderates the simple sugars of fruit so they provide us with lots of energy without large fluctuations in blood sugar.

I want you to eat fruit as dessert, snacks, and garnish for cereal. Fruit provides bulk to a meal and can make a light meal more filling. For example, a medium banana, which delivers 100 calories, contains no fat, little protein, and about 25 grams of carbohydrate. Bananas are so "rich" they seem to contain fat but don't, are pleasant to eat, and provide dietary fiber, vitamins, and minerals. Bananas are great by themselves, on cereal, in lowfat yogurt, as a flaming dessert, or as a simple snack.

Caution: Dried Fruit

Dried fruits by themselves are fine, but sometimes they are treated with the preservative sulfite. Sulfite can be detrimental to people with inflammatory problems, especially asthmatics. If you ever see it on an ingredients list or find it was used in processing—avoid the product. Vote with your pocketbook to eliminate unwanted additives and processing aids; the food industry will hear you.

Do: Other Fruits

"An apple a day keeps the doctor away" originated over eight hundred years ago in England. It was good advice then, and it's better advice today. Apples provide dietary fiber, minerals, vitamins, and satisfaction. But don't stop there. Also think peach, orange, pear, citrus fruits, banana, blueberries, blackberries, strawberries, watermelon, cantaloupe, melon, and on and on. Try them all, because unless your food diary says otherwise, they are good for you.

Canned fruit is generally canned in sugar syrup, which should be drained before use. If you can get fruit canned in its own juices, great; similarly for frozen fruit or fruit mixes. Simply read the ingredients list, and if it has sugar or corn syrup, don't use the product regularly.

Fruit Juice in Disguise

Fruit juices are okay if they are the whole juice. For example, fresh-squeezed orange juice or whole frozen orange juice is fine. So are apple, pear, apricot, prune, guava, pineapple, strawberry, peach, and other juices.

Don't use fruit juice unless it's the "natural" juice of the whole fruit. This means don't use clarified juice. Natural juices are usually cloudy because they contain the fiber and some starches. Drinks labeled fruit juice aren't always what you think. For example, read the ingredients list on a can of Hawaiian Punch. You will see it's about 10 percent juice and 90 percent various forms of sugar and flavors.

Caution: Fruit

Very rarely, some fruits will cause a reaction. You must experiment through the use of your food diary. Science simply doesn't have the answer, and there are no simple, valid tests. A thorough examination of all the medical literature has convinced me that personal experience is the best guide. And the value of fruit is so important that to rule out any class of fruit categorically would be wrong.

Suspect fruits include grapefruit, pineapple, and a few berries, such as blueberries and tomatoes. (Yes, tomatoes are berries.)

Fruits and Whole Juices: *Do's* for Arthritis Relief

Apples (all types)	Figs (all types)
Applesauce, unsweetened	Gooseberries
Apricots	Grapefruit
Bananas	Grapes (all types)
Blackberries	Guava
Blueberries	Honeydew melon
Boysenberries	Kiwifruit
Cantaloupe	Kumquats
Carambula	Lemons
Casaba melon	Loganberries
Cherries	Loquats
Cranberries	Lychees
Currants (all types)	Mangos
Dates (dried)	Mulberries
Elderberries	Nectarines

Oranges (all types)
Papayas
Passion fruit
Peaches
Pears
Persimmons
Pineapple
Plantains
Plums

Pomegranates
Prickly pears
Prunes
Raspberries
Sapodilla
Strawberries
Tangelos
Tangerines
Watermelon

Do Enjoy Nuts—But with Caution

I recommend nuts that are the "fruit" of a tree—walnuts, cashews, almonds, pecans, hazelnuts, pine nuts, and so on. But nuts, like fruit, must be subjected to testing. In general, they contain a great deal of fat, and generally they are heavily salted. If the salt isn't enough, artificial "smoke" flavor is often added. Read the ingredients list!

Remember, nuts contain alpha linolenic acid (ALA) that is desirable, and when nuts are used in recipes, their total calories are generally diluted, and they present a lesser concern.

Nuts Rated for Arthritis Relief (Omega-3 Oil Content)

Almonds (fair)
Cashews (good)
Chestnuts (excellent)
Litchi nuts (excellent)

Soybean nuts (good)
Walnuts (good, alpha linolenic acid)
Pine nuts (fair)

Do Take Supplements

The Arthritis Relief Diet makes use of sensible supplementation. The following are essential:

- *Multiple vitamin-mineral:* Take at least 50 percent of the RDI daily; 100 percent is fine. Review the supplements in chapter 12.
- *Calcium-magnesium:* Depending on your eating patterns, take at least 200 milligrams (and better still, 600 milli-

grams) of calcium in a supplement that also contains magnesium. If you're over 55, take 800 milligrams of calcium with magnesium. Be sure you always take your supplement at mealtime, because efficient absorption of calcium requires other food components, such as carbohydrates.

- *EPA:* Take at least three grams daily—five grams is better. Most EPA supplements contain 180 milligrams of EPA in each capsule; therefore, you should take six capsules daily as your insurance. To be certain, however, divide 1,000 by the number of milligrams of EPA in each capsule to obtain your daily number of capsules. For example, you would require three 360-milligram capsules, four 260-milligram capsules, or six 180-milligram capsules for one gram of EPA.
- *Flax oil:* Use as much as you can, either as capsules, or simply added to cereal, salads, and other foods. Don't use it in frying!
- Vitamin E: Take 100 to 400 I.U. daily.
- Vitamin C: Take at least one and preferably two 500-milligram doses daily.
- Fiber supplement: Take from three (10 percent of daily need) to 9 grams (30 percent of daily need) daily. Your fiber supplement should provide 3.5 to 4 grams of fiber per tablespoon. Ideally it will contain fiber from the following sources:
  Psyllium husks (mucilage)
  Apple fiber (pectin)
  Acacia gum (bile-acid elimination)
  Guar gum (bile-acid and fat elimination)
  Oat bran (cholesterol reduction)

Many good supplements contain only psyllium husks or are a purified psyllium extract. I recommend avoiding fiber supplements that contain cellulose or derivatives of it such as hydroxy methyl cellulose. Cellulose fiber "bulks" stools and improves regularity, but it does not absorb unwanted wastes and speed their elimination. And with all the excellent "natural" products available, there is simply no need for the cellulose products.

Now let's pause a moment and consider: About a thousand years ago when people worked hard and ate a diet rich in vegetables, they got about 80 grams of fiber daily. Technology, changes in food patterns, and modern life in general have reduced that to about 12 to 15 grams daily, and less for many people. Fiber is so important to our general health, and especially to arthritis relief, that I can't overemphasize its importance. I know you may be taking lots of supplements, and possibly some medication, and adding a fiber supplement might make you feel overwhelmed. The fact that fiber is natural and has absolutely no bad side effects should provide you with some encouragement. So, be encouraged that it's natural, will help you, and has absolutely no bad side effects.

Do Drink Lots of Water

You should consume four to eight glasses of water daily. Much of our water is consumed as other beverages, but if you resolve to drink at least four glasses of actual water, you will be helping to make your dietary fiber even more effective. And water will help your body eliminate unwanted metabolic by-products; that's sophisticated talk for waste materials.

Mineral water is an excellent beverage; you can't drink too much. Seek out one with lots of magnesium.

Do limit intake of coffee and other caffeine-containing beverages. The equivalent of two cups of coffee daily (about 150 to 200 milligrams) is sufficient caffeine without being excessive. Because decaffeinated coffee contains no caffeine, you can drink as much as you like.

Tea contains about 35 milligrams of caffeine per cup, so you can have four to six cups of tea without reaching your upper limit. An additional benefit of tea is that it's gentle on the stomach. Tea actually promotes stomach emptying and avoids an acid rebound. This is a special advantage if you are using aspirin or one of the aspirin derivatives for medication. Indeed, in my opinion, the beverage of choice for ulcer sufferers (often arthritics) is tea. And the best tea is standard black tea, such as Lipton or Tetley. One other factor in favor of tea is recent research showing it reduces heart disease and cancer to a small but perceptible degree.

In contrast to tea, coffee elicits an acid rebound. This means that when you drink several cups of coffee on an empty stomach, your stomach produces an excessive amount of acid and overshoots its mark, often creating an excessively acidic condition. This is not necessarily bad, because we usually don't drink coffee on an empty stomach. However, it doesn't help if you are using medication, such as aspirin or an aspirin derivative, that already has an effect on the stomach. If you're a coffee drinker, practice some moderation.

Occasionally enjoy soft drinks, but remember that if they are not artificially sweetened (diet drinks), they contain about seven teaspoons of sugar, and many also contain about 35 milligrams of caffeine per eight ounces. Better to choose from the wide variety of caffeine-free diet soft drinks available today.

Caution: Alcoholic Beverages

Wine can turn a good meal into a superb dining experience. Similarly, a cocktail can make an ordinary predinner discussion an elegant encounter. But when drinking alcohol, moderation should be the rule.

Although alcohol has never been proven to alter the course of inflammation, it does interact with some medications and often creates the potential for problems.

Excessive alcohol interferes with metabolism—specifically fat metabolism—and indirectly, that is what this dietary plan is all about. You see, to our body, alcohol is a deadly toxin; and the body's best defense is to metabolize it as quickly as possible. So when you drink, your body simply sets things aside and "burns up" the alcohol. Well, if you keep the alcohol coming, your body sets fat and sugar aside. Keep it up, and you've got fat deposits in your liver, as well as elevated blood sugar.

When you drink in moderation—say a cocktail before dinner or a glass or two of wine with dinner—your liver can handle it quite easily, and there is no problem. When you exceed that level, your liver is being overworked, even though you don't feel it. In addition, there is the detrimental effect on your brain or kidneys.

Indeed, a cocktail, a glass of wine, or beer with dinner is no problem. It only becomes a problem when excess prevails; so use caution and good judgment.

16

Menu Planning

This chapter translates the *Do's* and *Don'ts* into suggestions for breakfast, lunch, dinner, and snacks. The menu plans are based on interviews with individuals who have succeeded in controlling their arthritis with diet. They include people from many walks of life, such as teachers, secretaries, store clerks, management people, one corporation president, and a successful author. The self-employed include a doctor, a dentist, an acupuncturist, and several full-time mothers— the toughest profession of all. My hope is that you will see yourself or a loved one here and find ideas that fit your taste and lifestyle.

Breakfast: Getting Started

No matter how old you are or what you do in life, breakfast is your most important meal of the day. It will influence how you will feel all day (or night if you work nights)—so approach it with the respect it deserves.

Your objective at breakfast is to obtain complex carbohydrates, protein, and dietary fiber. Protein, necessary for all bodily processes, also helps maintain constant blood sugar, which helps eliminate mood swings.

Supplements

Morning is the ideal time to exercise (see chapter 18) and take your multiple vitamin-mineral supplement. It is also an excellent time to take EPA supplements, vitamins E and C, and supplemental fiber, if you do not eat a high-fiber breakfast and a daily diet rich in fish. Take high-fiber snacks during the day or a soluble fiber supplement in the evening.

Calcium supplements should always be taken with meals, as substances in food are essential for calcium absorption.

Breakfast Foods

Folk wisdom teaches you to always have "color on your plate." Breakfast should always include some fruit, which is an easy way to accomplish this requirement. Breakfast can be fruit alone—a fruit shake of fruit juice blended with a banana, melon, berries, or any combination you can devise. As unusual as it sounds, I've known people who blend cereals, including hot oatmeal, with apricot juice, flax oil, and some fruit into a breakfast shake.

Remember to apply the rules we've been building—use omega-3 oil and fiber, and emphasize *no* animal fat.

Fiber is one of the most important nutritional objectives of breakfast, and fruit can make a significant contribution. For example, most typical fruit servings supply from 1.5 to 5 grams of dietary fiber (five grams is about 20 percent of our daily need), and fruit fiber is excellent because much of it falls into the soluble category that helps remove waste materials from the system.

Fruit Juice

A morning glass of juice is enjoyed by people all over the world. When you choose juice, at least vow to drink genuine fruit juice. Frozen or canned is fine. Read the ingredients list and ask some questions. Does it contain only the juice of real fruit? If so, great. Does it contain sugar or corn syrup? If so, avoid it! Does it contain salt as one of the top three ingredients? If so, avoid it!

Fresh-squeezed is best. Remember, real juice is usually cloudy and often tastes somewhat bland. Orange juice, apple juice, tomato juice (also low-sodium V-8), prune juice, papaya juice, grapefruit juice, or pineapple juice should contain pulp and not be clear. And they're all excellent.

Cereal

Conduct a test. Take a piece of cereal and place it on your tongue with a lot of saliva. Swish it around for a few minutes. Is any significant residue left? If not, don't bother to eat it, because it's probably mostly sugar; if it leaves a good residue, it contains what you're after in a healthful cereal—fiber.

Next, conduct a reading test. Does the ingredients list state sugar or corn syrup before some real cereal—like corn? Is the sugar or corn syrup or both one of the first three ingredients? If so, don't use it!

Although I have not tested every cereal in this way, you may refer to chapter 15 for a list of many cereals that provide at least three grams of dietary fiber in a standard one-ounce serving.

I have discussed methods of preparing cereal with many people, and nothing surprises me. Oatmeal with apricot nectar was suggested by a woman who cannot use milk; I've tried it, and it is excellent.

Milk for Cereal, and for Coffee, Tea, and Drinking

I personally don't like skim milk because it seems watery and has a blue tinge; possibly it's my imagination, but so be it. There is a simple way to improve skim milk to make it taste better with a wholesome mouth feel: Simply add a few tablespoons of nonfat dry milk to a quart of skim milk. There's no exact amount, I simply put enough in to give it more taste and body. You can use it on cereal, in coffee or tea, and anywhere else you'd use milk. It's still fat-free—no arachidonic acid—tastes good, and has a higher protein delivery.

Eggs Versus Egg Beaters

You've made a commitment to health, but eggs may test your resolve. They do not fit directly into this diet. Egg substitutes are available, but beware—some contain more fat than eggs! Just remember to read the nutritional label.

My preferences are Egg Beaters or Scramblers. Both permit you to have scrambled eggs and omelets, which should include vegetables—especially zucchini, mushrooms, onions, chives, broccoli, spinach, and wheat germ. I have served nutritionists mushroom, onion, and garlic omelets made from Egg Beaters, and not one could tell that I didn't use eggs!

The addition of one ounce of skim-milk mozzarella cheese will add texture and body to the omelet. However, it is better to eat strictly vegetarian omelets without cheese.

Pancakes, Waffles, and French Toast

Pancakes and waffles can be made with the addition of unprocessed bran to add fiber; skim milk; Egg Beaters for eggs; and canola oil for shortening. The mix used should emphasize wheat or buckwheat flour as much as possible. Aunt Jemima mixes are my favorites, and they work fine with Egg Beaters.

Once the batter is prepared, spoon it onto the griddle and add sliced or diced fruit on top—especially berries (blueberries, raspberries, strawberries); but sliced peaches, apples, and bananas work equally well. Of course, you can also use fruit with waffles, but chop the fruit into small pieces and blend it with the batter.

French toast made with slightly dry sourdough bread, soaked in an Egg Beater batter using skim milk with some mild spice such as nutmeg or cinnamon, is excellent.

Topping for pancakes, waffles, and French toast should not include butter. The American classic, maple syrup, is excellent; but so is blueberry or boysenberry syrup, or some other natural syrup. Avoid the "glop" made from corn syrup, butter, and artificial flavor.

Other Possibilities for Breakfast

I enjoy watching people at breakfast in an international hotel's coffeeshop buffet. Most Americans head for the omelets, pancakes, waffles, bacon, and ham; a smaller number look to the cereals. People from Europe, Asia, and even Latin America commonly seek fish, beans and rice, vegetables, and even salad. However, all people seem to like fruit and fruit juice, and many take fried bananas, tomatoes, and onions.

Don't be a slave to habit. Be just as creative with breakfast as you are with other meals. Just maintain your omega-3 oil and other dietary objectives.

"Coffee Break"

Coffee is okay, tea is better, and juice better yet. More important is the "break snack." There should be no need for a snack, but that doesn't deter most people, so at least choose one that provides fiber and complex carbohydrate. If that sounds like fruit, it is! Don't eat doughnuts or sweet rolls; they elevate blood sugar only to let you down later. If you must eat something, make it a bran muffin. Remember, 18 percent of arthritics suffer from anxiety and depression— don't make it worse with bad snacking habits.

Lunch

Lunch is often the main meal of the day, but whatever the circumstances, it should accomplish several objectives:

1. EPA is a nutrient objective that can be obtained from fish (chapter 15) or as a supplement. Fish can be eaten as a tuna salad or sandwich, a nicely grilled swordfish steak, or even smoked trout. The only variables are lifestyle and economics. With a little imagination, fish can be eaten almost every day at lunch. With a little enthusiasm, some imagination, and willpower, lunch can get the bad fat out and the good EPA in.
2. Protein is always one major objective; indeed, it is often

the luncheon feature, especially in a restaurant. The protein can be obtained or enhanced as a garnish on pasta, the clams in a clam sauce, or shredded chicken over rice in a Chinese dish. There is no end to the variety.

3. Complex carbohydrate is important, especially the complex carbohydrate that comes so elegantly packaged by nature in rice, beans, vegetables, fruit, cereals, and grains (usually ending up in breads). This carbohydrate will provide the energy to carry you for the rest of the day and into the evening.

4. Dietary fiber, which is obtained from complex carbohydrate—especially in the grains and fruit—is also important.

5. Green leafy vegetables should, whenever possible, be part of every lunch. This is often obtained by the traditional green salad, which can consist of lettuce, spinach, watercress, sprouts, cabbage, and any other leafy vegetable. If you don't have a problem with them, tomatoes are excellent; if they are a problem, cucumbers and zucchini make good substitutes.

Power Lunches in a Blender

Soy protein isolates (the word "isolate" means the protein has been removed from the soy flour and has no soy oil, and very little carbohydrates) can be purchased as a protein mix that usually has the following nutritional delivery:

NUTRITION FACTS
Serving Size: 4 Rounded Tablespoons
(28.4g—approximately 1 heaping scoop)
Servings per container: 17

Amount Per Serving	Powder	Powder with 1 Cup Skim Milk
Calories	100	200
Calories from Fat*	0	8

Amount Per Serving	Powder	Powder with 1 Cup Skim Milk
	% Daily Value**	
Total Fat 0 g*	0%	2%
Saturated Fat 0 g	0%	2%
Cholesterol 0 mg	0%	2%
Sodium 200 mg	8%	14%
Potassium 200 mg	6%	20%
Total Carbohydrate 8 g	3%	7%
Dietary Fiber 0 g	0%	0%
Sugars 0 g		
Protein 16 g	30%	50%

Following will be a list of vitamins and minerals in the mix that provide from 20% to 130% of the RDI. If the one you purchase is similar, that is okay.

* Amount in Powder
** Percent Daily Values are based on a 2,000 calorie diet. Your daily values may be higher or lower depending on your calorie needs.

	Calories	2,000	2,500
Total Fat	Less than	65 g	80 g
Sat Fat	Less than	20 g	25 g
Cholesterol	Less than	300 mg	300 mg
Sodium	Less than	2,400 mg	2,400 mg
Total Carbohydrate		300 g	375 g
Dietary Fiber		25 g	30 g
Calories per gram:			

Fat 9   •   Carbohydrate 4   •   Protein 4

Blend this powder with a cup of orange juice or other nonsugared fruit juice and some fresh fruit such as a banana, strawberries, or an orange. You can also mix juice and milk (skim) for a more creamy texture. A lunch like this delivers excellent vegetable protein, no fat, and fruit fiber.

An advantage is derived from the vegetable protein, which supplies a generous portion of nonessential amino acids that your body will use for energy later. This provides stamina, the long-term energy that keeps you going when others are tired.

Afternoon Snacks

Snacking has become a worldwide pastime. You might as well join it. Snacks usually consist of carbohydrates of the wrong kind—empty-calorie sugar—so select those that would be healthy.

Popcorn is excellent; bran muffins, vegetable sticks, and fruit are all snacks that help you get a little closer to the objectives of this way of life you've chosen.

Tea or water is the best beverage. If you take soft drinks, use the low-calorie type; remember, the nondiet soft drinks contain about seven teaspoons of sugar per 12-ounce can.

Dinner

Dinner is traditionally the family gathering time, even in today's fast-paced world in which most people eat at least one and often two meals away from home. It is a chance to talk over the adventures and events of the day, to congratulate each other for a day well spent, and to search for solutions to the problems of today that will make a better tomorrow.

Such an important gathering must be an enjoyable event, and the menu selected should enhance the fellowship. Our health commitment can be shared by everyone, and all will be better for the experience. This plan is low in fat, low in cholesterol, and rich in those things that prevent heart disease and reduce the risk of cancer. Furthermore, the eating habits it instills in children will help them throughout life. Therefore, plan menus that everyone can enjoy.

Dinner is your final opportunity of the day to get EPA from food and not only as a supplement. But it is imperative that it not be one-sided—that it be appealing.

EPA is the major objective, but a secondary objective is to keep saturated fat to a minimum and polyunsaturated fat to a reasonable level. Thus the protein choice is important.

Main entrées for dinner can be as elaborate as you wish to make them. Trout stuffed with mushrooms, bread, onions, and scallions sautéed in olive oil laced with garlic is one of my favorites. But just as good is a piece of broiled frozen swordfish or a tuna salad without mayonnaise or with canola oil mayonnaise. If it's not fish, it can be as elaborate as pheasant, duck, guinea fowl, or simply breaded, skinned chicken (eat only the breast) sautéed in olive oil with a touch of garlic.

Dinner should always include a good source of complex carbohydrate such as rice, potato, Jerusalem artichoke, squash, carrots, wheat, corn, barley, or millet, and so on. Pasta is always excellent and can be the major part of the meal, including both protein and carbohydrate. Just don't overcook it; and serve it with a light sauce that includes chicken, clams, or some other high-protein source.

No dinner is complete without green vegetables, such as string beans, asparagus, broccoli, spinach, turnip greens, or other variations. Finally, a salad should accompany the menu. For a unique treat, try a carrot and cabbage salad that delivers a cruciferous vegetable as well as carrots. Cruciferous vegetables—broccoli, cabbage, cauliflower, Brussels sprouts, and so on—are especially healthy and have materials that help prevent cancer and heart disease. A rule in our house is that we have one serving of a cruciferous vegetable daily.

No dinner is complete without dessert—the tradition of many cultures. It has always been the children's reward associated with clearing the plate; and by the time we're adults, it's habit—something we expect. Nutritionally it often provides calcium in cheese or a fermented milk product.

Many desserts can be made or purchased that are completely acceptable on this plan. Fruit is the most natural and obviously acceptable and is excellent for this plan. Fruit pies and pumpkin and sweet potato pies are all fine. Common sense dictates that cream pies are not good because they contain sources of arachidonic acid.

Cakes are not good choices for dessert, as they are usually somewhat high in fat. However, an occasional small portion is not a problem.

Ice Cream

Ice cream seems to be a favorite dessert for many. You can purchase ice cream that is nonfat. This means you can enjoy a universally accepted treat without the consequences. And you can always select sherbet—with no fat, naturally.

You are trying to avoid butter and egg yolks, although in most ice cream recipes these components are diluted over many servings. And there are basic recipes that can include margarine, Egg Beaters, and olive oil; in which case you're home free.

Ten Days—Ten Menus

The following menus were created by people who have gained control of their arthritis. With these meals—and variations that you can create, using part 1 of this book and following the *Do's* and *Don'ts* of chapter 15—you can begin to feel better too.

D A Y 1

This sample menu came to me from a 42-year-old mother with arthritis who cooks for her husband and children. They pull together with her, and they are better and healthier for the commitment.

Breakfast:

- Pancakes made with Aunt Jemima buckwheat pancake and waffle mix and skim milk, Egg Beaters, Puritan oil, and ½ cup unprocessed bran; she adds a sliced apple to each pancake immediately after pouring the batter on the griddle.
- Maple syrup—the real kind.
- Orange juice; coffee with nondairy creamer.
- Bran muffins.

Lunch:

- Barbecued chicken; charcoal-barbecued breasts and legs with the skin removed, using barbecue sauce. For other members of the family, skin is left on while barbecuing.

- Three-bean salad, using green, waxed, and kidney beans marinated in Wish-Bone Italian dressing with onions, crushed garlic clove, and oregano.
- Salad made with lettuce, shaved carrots, sliced zucchini, and green peppers.
- Steamed asparagus.
- Fruit salad made with apples, strawberries, melon, and diced pineapple.
- Beer (one glass).
- Coffee.

Dinner:

- Broiled salmon—pink, juicy, and slightly browned.
- Long-grain rice with parsley and shallots.
- Sliced zucchini sautéed in olive oil with mushrooms and onions.
- Tuna salad sandwich for son who wouldn't eat salmon.
- Apple pie.

Supplements:

- Multiple vitamin-mineral: One tablet.
- Calcium: Three totaling 600 milligrams.
- EPA: Four capsules.
- Flax oil: Add one tablespoon to "three bean salad."
- A fiber supplement.
- Vitamin E: 400 I.U.
- Vitamin C: 500 milligrams.

D A Y   2

From a 33-year-old nonworking mother of two children, aged 11 and 8; she developed arthritis at age 32. She prepares the same meals for everyone.

Breakfast:

- Oatmeal with zanta currants. She uses skim milk and sugar on her oatmeal, with one tablespoon of flax oil. Her husband and children use lowfat milk.
- Grapefruit.
- Coffee.

Mid-morning:

- Hot tea with an apple or pear.

Lunch:

- Tuna chunks with canola oil and a spoonful of flax oil and lemon juice mixed with chopped celery, served over a half avocado on top of a lettuce leaf.
- Sourdough bread.
- Iced tea.
- Melon balls topped with strawberry yogurt.
- Coffee or tea with oatmeal cookies.

Dinner:

- Spinach spaghetti with tomato sauce containing shaved carrots, sliced mushrooms (sautéed in olive oil with garlic), onions, oregano, and basil.
- Lettuce and tomato salad with sliced red peppers, zucchini, tomatoes, and asparagus chunks; Wish-Bone Caesar salad dressing with one spoonful of flax oil.
- Strawberries over pound cake, topped with strawberry yogurt.
- Hot tea.

Supplements:

- Multiple vitamin-mineral: One tablet at breakfast.
- Calcium: Two tablets at lunch and dinner.
- EPA: Three capsules.
- Fiber: One tablespoon of store brand psyllium.
- Flax oil: One tablespoon.

D A Y 3

Created by a woman, age 45, who works as a seamstress in a shop that makes seat covers of canvas and other heavy-duty materials. Manual dexterity is essential to her job. She has two children, 4 and 16.

Breakfast:

- All-Bran with skim milk and sliced banana. The rest of the family has other cereal and uses lowfat milk.
- Prune juice. Other family members have orange juice.
- Coffee.

Lunch:

- A brown bag lunch, consisting of a sliced turkey breast sandwich with pita bread, Wish-Bone blue cheese dressing, and a sliced avocado.
- Apple and carrot sticks or other fruit.
- Coffee.

Morning and Afternoon Break:

- Bran muffin and coffee.

Dinner:

- Baked burrito with beans, onions, peppers, and sour cream. The children had a fried ground-beef burrito.
- Rice with tomato sauce containing small cubes of green pepper.
- Barbecued chicken breast.
- Loganberry pie (baked from frozen Mrs. Smith's).

Supplements:

- Multiple vitamin-mineral: two tablets.
- Calcium: three 200-milligram tablets.

- EPA: six tablets.
- Vitamin E: 400 I.U.
- Vitamin C: 500 milligrams.

DAY 4

From an executive secretary, 50 years old, with two grown children. She and her husband, a real-estate manager, use her earnings to travel extensively on vacations. Her arthritis appeared as morning stiffness and swollen fingers. She had her rings made larger before she started the diet plan. After three months her fingers were normal, and she had no morning stiffness or joint aches.

Breakfast:

- Fiber One cereal with skim milk, sliced strawberries, and one tablespoon of flax oil.
- Orange juice.
- Half grapefruit.

Lunch:

- Salad purchased in cafeteria, consisting of lump salmon in a large, hollowed-out tomato with lots of lemon and shredded lettuce.
- Sliced apple.
- Hot tea with lemon.

Morning and Afternoon Snacks:

- Fiber wafers.
- Tea (one cup in the morning and one in the afternoon).

Dinner:

- Baked breaded chicken (skin removed before breading).

- Rice, boiled and mixed with sautéed vegetables, spiced with oregano.
- Vegetables (asparagus slices, zucchini, mushroom slices, onion, and garlic clove) sautéed in olive oil.
- Small salad of lettuce and cucumber with Italian dressing.
- Orange sherbet with sliced oranges.

Supplements:

- Multiple vitamin-mineral: one tablet.
- Calcium: 600 milligrams daily.
- EPA: two capsules.
- Vitamin E: 400 I.U.
- Vitamin C: 500 milligrams twice daily.
- Fiber: store brand fiber supplement.

DAY 5

An "executive." He is 40 years old, and his arthritis was diagnosed four years ago. The diet, together with his doctor's support, has helped him reduce medication use. In addition, his general health, especially his heart, has improved on this plan. He is married with three children; they are a tennis family who enjoy outdoor activities. His wife prepares and follows this diet also.

Breakfast:

- Oatmeal with raisins and skim milk.
- Melon.
- Juice (usually orange).

Lunch:

- Broiled salmon (or "fish of the day") with rice and broccoli at a local restaurant with coworkers. They had wine—he had iced tea.

Dinner:

- Rainbow trout (frozen) sautéed with garlic in olive oil and stuffed with bread chunks and mushrooms.
- Cooked corn (frozen).
- String beans.
- Carrot and cabbage salad.
- Dessert of lemon chiffon pie.
- Chardonnay.

Supplements:

- Multiple vitamin-mineral: one tablet at breakfast.
- Calcium: one tablet at dinner.
- Fiber: vegetable fiber supplement (generic).
- EPA: one capsule
- Flax oil: on cereal

D A Y   6

An active, 14-year-old girl who was stricken with arthritis at age 12. Her family supports her with this dietary commitment. The reinforcement by the family—brothers and sisters—is essential. She is under close medical supervision and on medication. The Arthritis Relief Diet allowed her doctor to cut back her medication.

Breakfast:

- Oatmeal with raisins, skim milk, and brown sugar.
- One half grapefruit.

Lunch: (Brown bag to school)

- Sandwich: Tuna salad on pita bread with lettuce and avocado (no tomato).
- Apple, sliced for easy eating.
- Oatmeal cookies.
- Packaged orange drink made from juice.

Snack:

- Popcorn made in microwave—no butter or salt.

Dinner:

- Chicken Mango, using skinless chicken breast sliced and sautéed, then cooked briefly with mango and lemon slices.
- Brown long-grain rice.
- String beans (French cut), broccoli, and pearl onions.
- Strawberry chiffon pie with sliced strawberries.

Supplements:

- Multiple vitamin-mineral: one tablet at breakfast.
- Calcium: two tablets at dinner.
- EPA: three capsules before bedtime (otherwise they cause an aftertaste for her).
- Vitamin E: 400 I.U. every other day.
- Vitamin C: 500 milligrams daily.

D A Y 7

From a mother of three teenagers who's married to an active, outdoors-oriented husband. She has learned to control arthritis completely by diet. This sample is from a Saturday when the entire family eats together.

Breakfast:

- Waffles (made with Aunt Jemima mix, unprocessed bran, Egg Beaters, and blueberries); flax oil added to the batter; maple syrup.
- Bran muffin with coffee.

Lunch:

- Barbecued tuna steaks (purchased frozen; thawed in a microwave prior to cooking on the charcoal grill).

- Salad with chunks of lettuce, celery, zucchini, carrots, green peppers, and cucumbers.
- Sliced peaches with yogurt.

Dinner:

- Chicken cut in short strips and cooked quickly in a wok, using peanut oil and garlic.
- Wok-cooked vegetables with pineapple chunks: asparagus (sliced diagonally), water chestnuts, sliced zucchini, and grated cabbage. (The chicken is served on top of the vegetables with the pineapple chunks, which are cooked last. The entire dish is served over rice; soy sauce used if desired.)

Supplements:

- Multiple vitamin-mineral: three tablets daily.
- Calcium: three 250-milligram tablets.
- EPA: three capsules.
- Flax oil: on salads.

D A Y 8

From a 65-year-old midwestern homemaker whose arthritis has been with her since she was about 40. By experimenting with this and other dietary approaches, she has increased her mobility (she bicycles), has been able to maintain reduced inflammation, and uses medication only as necessary (an occasional NSAID). Both she and her husband keep their weight down. She has identified foods to which she is sensitive, and they both simply avoid them. She enjoys cooking.

Breakfast:

- Oatmeal with fruit, lowfat yogurt, and wheat germ. She especially likes blueberry yogurt this way. Thus the cereal can be eaten like a classic Bavarian muesli,

a German breakfast food prepared by mixing whole grains with yogurt, nuts, berries, and pieces of fruit.
* Bran muffins with prune chunks added before cooking.
* Coffee with nondairy creamer.

Lunch:

* Red cabbage, onions, and long sliced carrots sautéed in canola oil.
* Lightly sautéed chicken strips served with the cabbage and onions.
* Tea.

Dinner:

* Frozen fish fillet breaded after thawing by dipping in an egg white and skim milk mix and then coating with a mixture of flour, dried bread crumbs, and parsley.
* Vegetables—lightly steamed broccoli served with boiled white rice.
* Apple cake (similar to a pie, but without a crust).
* Tea for her; coffee for him.

Supplements:

* Multiple vitamin-mineral: one tablet in the morning and one in the evening.
* Calcium: three capsules, one at each meal, totalling 600 milligrams daily.
* Vitamin C: one 500-milligram tablet daily.
* EPA: four taken at bedtime.

DAY 9

From a 55-year-old woman who chairs an arthritis support group. Members of this group meet monthly to help each other cope by sharing things that work.

These meals are to some extent an outcome of their participation. She has found from her food diary that she cannot use milk or tomatoes, and she has devised recipes that many have adopted.

Breakfast:

- Oatmeal muesli: cooked oatmeal mixed with apricot nectar, a generous portion of wheat germ, and raisins. Oatmeal can be cooked slowly in the apricot nectar as well.

Lunch:

- Pasta salad.
- Tea or coffee.
- Fruit.

Dinner:

- Japanese-style (flavored with a soy-based sauce) fish steaks.
- Red cabbage—a high-fiber vegetable dish.
- Mushroom rice.
- Apple cake.

Snacks:

- Popcorn—no butter, moderate salt.

Supplements:

- Multiple vitamin-mineral: one tablet at breakfast and one at dinner.
- Calcium: four tablets for 800 milligrams daily.
- Vitamin C: 500 milligrams daily.
- Vitamin E: 400 I.U. every other day.
- EPA: three capsules.
- Fiber supplement.

D A Y   10

Our final menus come from a 50-year-old real-estate saleswoman who often puts in 12-hour days, seven days a week, during the "high" season.

Breakfast:

- All-Bran cereal with banana slices and skim milk.
- Coffee.

Mid-morning Snack:

- Coffee.

Lunch:

- Fish stew or fish in a restaurant.
- Iced tea made from instant mix.

Dinner:

- Herb fish (fish broiled with a blending of spices and herbs that impart flavor).
- Braised peas with lettuce.
- Minute Rice.
- Apple cake.

Supplements:

- Multiple vitamin-mineral: one tablet in the morning and one in the evening.
- Calcium: two tablets (one in the morning and one in the evening).
- EPA: three capsules daily.
- Fiber snacks during the day.

Dining Out

I had a call from a woman on this diet. "Dr. Scala, it's our anniversary, and we're going out to dinner; can I go off the diet for one night?"

To me that's no problem, but they live in the Midwest, where eating out means eating beef. I played dumb. "Why is it necessary to go off the diet?" I queried.

"Well, because I know that my husband will want a steak, and I'm sure that's what I'll want also."

The conversation slowly changed when I learned that they would be going to a rather expensive restaurant; in fact, the restaurant served live Maine lobsters—expensive, but fine for this diet. I urged her to try a lobster—it would be an adventure for her, while she gave her husband a night off from her diet, so to speak.

A few months later I had a follow-up call from this woman. She and her husband had started a ritual of eating out two or three times a month. As she put it: "We both get a night off—I don't have to cook, my husband gets a chance to eat something other than my diet, and it's added some spice to our lives. You were right, Dr. Scala, I can eat out and still follow my diet. Thanks for your encouragement."

Dining out affords an opportunity to try new things, and to give the people around us an opportunity to eat something different. All you have to do is follow the *Do's* and *Don'ts.*

Assert yourself by telling your waiter that you are on a special diet, and if you see something on the menu that looks good, ask questions. For example, in an Italian restaurant ask if they have a nonmeat sauce, or if their clam sauce is light, without cream. Can sole *meuniére* be prepared in olive oil, not butter? The possibilities become endless if you're willing to ask questions and assert your role—that of the customer!

Most chefs can prepare excellent vegetarian meals, and frozen fish is available everywhere. If you think fresh fish is always available, let me describe an experience I had while at a meeting of the Nutrition Foundation.

We were eating at an expensive restaurant that emphasized seafood. Since it was in Florida, and they had scrod (a cold-water fish) as the day's special, I asked the waitress: "How do you get fresh scrod in Naples, Florida?"

Her reply startled everyone who had been extolling the excellent fresh fish: "None of our fish is fresh; it's all selected as fresh, frozen at sea."

Since then I've spoken to many people who fish for a hobby and freeze what they catch because it gives the fish "a better texture," in their words.

Beyond the entrée, the rest is easy, because it's vegetables, rice, fruit, and salad—all things that are on the *Do* list.

Breakfast out is usually the major problem meal. That's because we Americans seem locked into eggs, bacon, and sausage. But in many restaurants, pancakes, waffles, cereal, fruit, toast, and even fish are often on the menu. Remember, the amount of egg yolk you get in a serving of pancakes or waffles is not really important. But you must exercise will-power over the meat (such as sausage or bacon).

Many restaurants make Egg Beaters omelets or even an egg white omelet. More and more restaurants are leaning toward dishes recommended by the American Heart Association. These dishes, marked on the menu with a healthy heart symbol, are usually low in animal fat and generous in complex carbohydrate and are good sources of protein. Still other restaurants are offering "health" menus that emphasize fish, vegetables, and lighter, yet filling dishes.

Call before you go and ask what's available.

The following is a progress report to use when you are a few months into your new diet. Make notes now—impression, questions, what you think will be the most difficult part of your diet—then see how far you've come.

Six-Month Progress Report

Proactions

On a lined piece of paper, answer the following questions:

- Have I eliminated as much animal fat from my diet as humanly possible? (For example, cut out meat, fat-containing dairy products, etc.?)

- Have I taken flax oil (up to 45 grams daily) and/or EPA (three or more grams daily)?
- Have I taken a multiple vitamin-mineral supplement daily?
- Have I kept a food diary to identify foods that trigger my flare-ups?

Better Health

- How am I feeling?
- Do I have more or less morning stiffness?
- Do I have more or less swollen and painful joints?
- Am I able to do more activities than when I started the New Arthritis Relief Diet?
- Has my outlook improved?
- Is my doctor supportive? If yes, great! If no, ask yourself, "Did I show him/her the book and point out the medical references?" If yes to this question, have you consulted with another doctor?

IV

Thriving Versus Surviving

You have come a long way. You have gained new insight into controlling your illness and gaining control over your life. That is just common-sense survival, and it puts you in the "above average" category. Now you are ready to move to the "head of the class."

Thriving means that you will have control over every aspect of your life. Sure, it develops slowly, and you might never notice it happening; but your body will soon be running smoothly. Your appearance will improve, and people will notice. Most important, your inner strength will grow as you gain the inner joy that can only come to those who make the most of life.

17

How to Lose Weight Naturally

All arthritis experts agree on one point: People who have arthritis should not be overweight. Common sense, if not experience, tells you that your weight-bearing joints—knees, hips, and ankles—hurt more, and restrict your activity more, if you are overweight. What you learn by experience and intuition every expert confirms.

Excessive weight aggravates the non-weight-bearing joints as well. In fact, the entire arthritic condition goes into a downward spiral with a weight increase, and as this continues, the arthritis gets worse. It's a behavior-related pattern, not part of arthritis itself.

As arthritis begins, activity decreases and anxiety increases—which usually leads to frustration. Many of us then relieve our frustrations by eating processed foods. Obviously, eating adds weight, and these convenience foods are usually high in calories. The weight comes on slowly at first, then more rapidly as activity decreases. Worse, is the excessive weight makes the arthritis more intense, and the cycle of overeating and underexercising continues.

To add insult to injury, arthritis makes cooking more difficult. Let's face it, aching hands are not able to manipulate pots and pans; and standing over a stove brings aches to sore knees. It's easier to eat convenience foods, which are more fattening, less nutritious, and—when compared to the foods I recommend—totally inadequate.

Weight Management Is Essential in Arthritis

No health challenge is simpler nor more difficult than achieving and maintaining your desirable weight. By age 45, most people would like to shed about 10 pounds, and lots do; but within a year or so, the weight is usually back on—plus a few extra pounds. Some surveys show that 74 percent of North American adults are overweight. Many adults who face this modern dilemma just give up and go through life overweight, which isn't healthy.

Why Is Weight So Important?

Being overweight is bad for you! Excess body fat increases the risk of developing most cancers by about 45 percent and increases the risks of heart disease, high blood pressure, and diabetes by about 30 percent. Excess weight makes arthritis and any other inflammatory autoimmune disease worse and, when compared to normal or slightly underweight people, shortens life by about 20 percent.

In contrast, extensive research following people for more than 20 years has proven that if overweight people with arthritis lose weight, the arthritis improves and they live longer. Moreover, the people who lost weight escaped adult onset diabetes and their mortality declined by 20 percent; cancer and heart disease rates returned to their age-related normal. In summary, losing weight and keeping it off pays big dividends in more ways than only helping arthritis.

Why Do I Gain Weight So Easily?

Weight gain is driven by basic evolutionary and physiological forces that work in one direction only: more body fat.

The first force is survival. Your body has the ability to store excess calories as fat; in our distant past, those extra calories kept us alive when food was scarce. Extra body fat made long sea voyages possible and got people through prolonged droughts. Indeed, even today a somewhat heavy, but not obese, person survives cancer chemotherapy better than a slim person.

The second factor is our body's efficiency. When you were young and lean, you burned more calories just to keep your body running, as you'll see when I discuss basal metabolism. Your basal metabolism declines as you age, as do the calories you need to stay alive and even perform daily tasks. Conversely, eating habits (along with personality) are established during youth, and unless you change them, you go on eating the same amount of food. In fact, you usually eat more food, since it relates to increased social interaction. Thus, we need fewer calories as we get older, but we actually get more and burn even less.

The third force is our social structure. No longer scarce for most people, food has become a major part of daily life. In any large urban area it's all around us in advertising, fast-food outlets, and various exotic food stores and vendors. Even when we are out in the country we are seldom 30 minutes from a meal or snack. Worse, fast foods are usually the most fattening.

The fourth force is today's complex lifestyle. Social pressure, work, and family stress drive you to eat more than you should. Other things, such as deception in the form of "low-fat" or "low-calorie" foods, "business" meals, travel, and family and social gatherings all lead you to eat more food. The worst stress is boredom, which drives many of us to watch TV with a numb mind but active taste buds. Exercise is the best stress outlet, yet most people tend to eat because it's easier and more sociable.

Now see how simple it is to gain or lose an extra pound.

Losing Weight Is Simple

A pound of fat represents about 3,500 calories. Create a 3,500-calorie deficit, and you will lose about one pound; conversely, eat an extra 3,500 calories, and you'll gain a pound. It's like a bank balance: add extra money and your account grows; remove money and it shrinks. So an extra 10 pounds is a calorie surplus of about 35,000 calories. Conversely, to lose 10 pounds you have to create a deficit of 35,000 calories. Isn't that arithmetic simple?

For example, suppose you did everything exactly the same each day but cut out 350 calories of food or burned an extra 350 calories as exercise. A dessert is usually about that much—or you could simply cut about 100 calories out of each meal and not use sugar and cream in your coffee or tea. In 10 days you'd create a 3,500-calorie deficit, and after a hundred days you would be 10 pounds lighter. Sound simple? It's not!

In my example I said, "Do everything exactly the same." You might think you are, but your body has some tricks that it uses to save those extra survival calories. Your body can lower basal metabolism just a little and spend a few less calories here and there that you won't notice. We call this weight defense the "set point," because once you've been at a weight for some time, your body tries to stay at that weight or even gain a little more for safety. It is as if your body is saying, "I like it here and want to survive, so don't mess around. And while I'm at it, I'll gain a little for insurance." Determination can overcome that set point.

We don't live so precisely that we can cut exactly 350 calories a day. In fact, on a cool day we need more calories and on a hot day less, as temperature control is part of our basal metabolism. Walk one day, ride the next, use an elevator, sleep an extra hour, and the whole idea of "exactly the same" goes up in smoke. Therefore, you really need to create a bigger deficit to start weight loss going and even to keep it going.

Basal Metabolism and Activity: How Many Calories Do You Burn?

Most daily energy is used by your body to manage its many functions. We call this the basal metabolic rate (BMR); it represents the number of calories you need daily to maintain temperature, blood flow, urine production, breathing, and virtually everything your body does, including thinking. A good way to visualize basal metabolism is to think of it as the energy you'd burn if you just sat in bed all day. Interestingly, your brain uses a large block of energy whether you use it or not. Much mental activity goes to managing body functions, while thinking only adds a modest amount.

Calculate Your Basal Metabolic Rate

Women

You can easily calculate your BMR using a pocket calculator. For example:

For a 120-pound, 5′4″, 35-year-old woman:

Basic level:		= 655
4.36 × weight in pounds:	4.36 × 120	= 523.2
4.32 × height in inches (5′4″):	4.32 × 64	= 276.5
Total		1454.7
Subtract 4.7 × age	4.7 × 35	− 164.5
Calories		= 1290.2

Basal metabolism is 1,290 calories per day.

The basic level (655) is a factor that applies to all women; it was derived by measuring thousands, if not millions, of women. The factor 4.36 accounts for the calories necessary to keep all your organs working, based on your weight. The next factor (4.32) times height accounts for your body surface area and the calories lost to either keep you warm or cool, as the case may be. The factor 4.7, which is practically the same for everyone, times your age accounts for the decline in BMR as you get older.

How Many Calories Do You Use in a Typical Day?

Take our 120-pound woman again:

Activity Level	Multiplier*	Calories
Light activity in sedentary person: (Sits most of day; e.g., secretary, clerk, executive)	1.3 × BMR =	1,677
Moderately active: (Exercises three to four times weekly, 30 minutes per session, and walks to various places)	1.4 × BMR =	1,806
Active in exercise and daily activity: (Exercises more than four times weekly, 30–40 minutes per session)	1.6 × BMR =	2,064
Exceptionally active: (Exercises six times weekly, 40 minutes per session; walks a lot and enjoys sports)	1.8 × BMR =	2,322

* The multiplier is derived by extensive research on people who are active to various levels. These are quite accurate if a person is honest about her level of activity.

How would an overweight 5′4″, 36-year-old woman, who weighs 140 pounds, achieve 125 pounds?

Her BMR is (round to nearest whole number):

$655 + (4.36 × 140) + (4.32 × 64) − (4.7 × 36) = 1,373$ calories

If she is moderately active, her daily calorie use is:

$1.4 × BMR = 1,922$

A 1,000-calorie diet would create a daily deficit of 922 calories. If her target is 125 pounds, her goal is clear:

15 pounds × 3,500 = 52,500 calories ÷ 922 = 57 days

It would take about two months of a 1,000-calorie daily diet while maintaining a moderately active life, to achieve her target weight.

This is a very realistic objective. When she achieves her 125-pound goal, her eating pattern should fit the following level:

BMR: 655 + (4.36 × 125) + (4.32 × 64) − (4.7 × 36) = 1,307 calories
Maintain a moderately active lifestyle: 1.4 × BMR = 1,830 calories

If she maintains a modest exercise program and eats sensibly, she will easily maintain 125 pounds. At 1,830 calories, it is difficult even for a dietitian to eat a truly balanced diet, so I emphasize again the importance of sensible supplementation with a multiple vitamin-mineral supplement, calcium, fiber, and—to manage arthritis—EPA and flax oil.

Men

For a 6′0″, 26-year-old man who weighs 180 pounds:

Basic level:		=	66.0
6.22 × weight in pounds:	6.22 × 180	=	1,119.6
12.7 × height in inches (6′0″):	12.7 × 72	=	914.4
Total		=	2,100.0
Subtract 6.8 × age:	6.8 × 26	−	176.8
Calories		=	1,923.2

Basal metabolism is 1,923 calories per day.

Daily Calorie Use

Activity Level	Multiplier	Calories
Sedentary:	1.3 × BMR	= 2,500
(Light activity)		
Moderately active:	1.4 × BMR	= 2,692
Very active:	1.6 × BMR	= 3,077
Exceptional:	1.8 × BMR	= 3,461

How would an overweight, 6′0″, 36-year-old man, who weighs 210 pounds, achieve 185 pounds?

I meet many men in this predicament. You can usually spot them by their bulging waistlines.

His BMR is (rounded up):

$66 + (6.22 \times 210) + (12.7 \times 72) - (6.8 \times 36) = 2,042$

If he is moderately active, his daily calorie use is:

$1.4 \times BMR = 2,858.8$

This man now has a clear target for a healthy weight.

Exercise: A "No Brainer"

Obviously, if you are willing to increase your calorie output with exercise, you can speed the weight-loss process by 10 percent. In addition, exercise will increase muscle and bone mass (remember your calcium), which is more compact, smooth, and attractive than fat. Muscle and bone weigh more than fat, so as you exercise, your target weight can shift slightly upward—and you'll still be happy with the results.

BMR and Age: We Really Do Get Better As We Age!

We really *do* improve with age: As our body learns to do things more efficiently with age, our BMR declines. The following tabulation illustrates this point using a typical woman and man at various ages. Let's agree that they are both moderately active people. I used our calculation for this; why not do it for yourself and get a feeling for how much energy you will use.

BMR and Age

Age	Woman 5'6", 130 pounds	Man 6'0", 190 pounds
	Calories	*Calories*
25	1,947	2,789
35	1,889	2,694
45	1,814	2,598
55	1,749	2,503
65	1,683	2,408

The difference between a 25-year-old and a 65-year-old is 14 percent in calories expended on a daily basis. Slowing down in external activity, such as sports, as we get older, probably causes the difference to be more like 30 percent. That wouldn't be so bad if our eating habits didn't become established so early and social pressures didn't increase eating. Basic eating habits are firmly established by age 25, and they only change if we consciously work at changing them for the better. That's another reason why you're using this book.

I've heard all the excuses:

"If there's no beef, it's not a meal."

"When I don't have dessert, I don't feel like I finished my meal."

"All I heard as a child was about the starving children in India. I still clean whatever is on my plate, including dessert."

"Breakfast meant bacon or sausage. Every Sunday it also meant home fries."

"I always had a sweet roll with my coffee at ten-thirty and again at three."

"Spaghetti isn't right without meatballs or an Italian sausage."

"Every Saturday we had two hot dogs at lunch. If I don't now, I feel something is missing."

Get the point? These eating patterns are established when you are young and become part of your personality. It takes a little effort, but they can be changed for the better, much like other behavioral traits. It's all about setting goals.

Why Diets Don't Work

Folk wisdom teaches, "You cannot run away from your problems because you have to take yourself along." Weight control is that way as well. Sure, you can lose the weight by the plan I will describe shortly, but the factors that caused your overweight usually remain unchanged in spite of your accomplishment. Research has proven that unless people develop new eating and exercise habits they usually put back on more weight than they lost. Let's examine some habits that research has proven work.

Proven Habits That Keep Weight Off

Cultivate these habits, nurture them, and you will keep your weight at the desirable level.

- Eat for bulk. A large piece of fruit or a vegetable and a square of chocolate have about the same calories. You can swallow the chocolate in a gulp and remain hungry. Eat the fruit or vegetable slowly, and you won't be hungry. Always select food for bulk and think "vegetarian" whenever you sit down to eat!
- Eat at least two meals daily. Chew your food carefully, and put your eating utensils down between each bite; don't pick them up until you have swallowed the food. Extensive research has proven this careful eating behavior helps people lose weight. It works because the feeling of fullness (satiety) usually lags behind your rate of eating. So slow down your eating rate, and your brain has a chance to help you eat less.
- Avoid all fried food.
- Avoid sauces and gravies.
- Use meat as a garnish or condiment over something bulky like rice; never eat fried meat or meat with sauce.
- Have at least two vegetables and some fruit at each meal.
- Have fruit for dessert with no syrup or whipped cream.
- Drink a full glass of water 15 to 30 minutes before each meal; take a fiber supplement at that time. Taking fiber 30 minutes before a meal makes you feel "full."
- Snack on vegetables or fruit only!

The Seven-Day, Quick-Loss Diet

We put weight on slowly, but we want to get it off quickly. With that in mind, I've devised a plan that works well, doesn't compromise your health, and will take about 5 percent of your weight off in a week to 10 days. I call it the Alternate Diet Plan.

An Alternate-Day Liquid Diet Plan

It's simple. One day use the soy protein powder supplement described in chapter 16, mixed in juice or nonfat milk as I described. Take it four times, preceded by a fiber supplement, as I've discussed. The next day, apply sensible eating habits, or eat one complete meal with fish and two protein powder meals. Doing this on alternate days works because it's easy to control, and you get to eat!

Summary of Alternate-Day Diet Plan

I am not an advocate of quick weight-loss programs or gimmick diets. However, the Alternate Diet Plan will cause weight to come off quickly; you'll be on your way. Then switch to the regular Arthritis Relief Diet, and keep the weight loss going.

Remember, you need about 65 grams of protein daily to repair, rebuild, and meet normal body needs; very few extra protein calories are converted to fat.

What Is a "K Cal"?

A calorie is the very small amount of energy necessary to raise a gram of water one degree in temperature. Scientists have long expressed calories in increments of 1,000 at a time. Since kilo means "one thousand," we actually express the calories in food as kilocalories. However, the *kilo* (abbreviated as "K") is usually left off and the word *calorie* is capitalized. I use K cal here for accuracy, but remember that most of the time you see the word *calorie*, capitalized or not, it usually means kilocalories.

Low-Calorie Day

Three Times Daily:

Soy protein powder mixed in juice (no sugar added)   600 K cal.
or nonfat milk.

20 to 30 minutes before protein drink:
Take a fiber supplement mixed in water *or*   None
Take a fiber supplement mixed in juice.   210 K cal.

Total: **810 K cal.**

If you take fiber in water, you have two options:
Eat three vegetable snacks, or one piece of fruit   200 K cal.
divided in half for two snacks.

Total: **800 K cal.**

Additional supplements:
Multiple vitamin-mineral: two tablets.
Calcium-magnesium: three tablets for 600 milligrams of calcium.
Vitamin C: 500 milligrams.
Vitamin E + selenium: one capsule.
EPA: three capsules.
Flax oil: add a tablespoon in protein mix (use blender).

Low-Calorie Day with Food

Breakfast and Lunch:
Two meals: Protein powder in juice or nonfat milk.   400 K cal.
Snacks:
Two vegetable snacks.   200 K cal.
Fiber Supplements (three times a day):
Take a fiber supplement mixed in water before   None
each meal.
Dinner:
One light meal: salad with lots of lettuce; grated   250 K. cal.
carrots; and 3½ ounces (100 grams) broiled
or baked fish.

Total: **850 K cal.**

Supplements:

Multiple vitamin-mineral: two tablets.
Calcium-magnesium: 600 milligrams total.
Vitamin C: 500 milligrams.
Vitamin E + selenium: 400 I.U. + 50 micrograms (one capsule).
EPA: three capsules.
Flax oil: one tablespoon in protein mix.

Seven-Day Diet Plan

1st Day: Low-calorie day (three or four protein powder meals).

2nd Day: Low-calorie day with food (two protein powder meals, one light meal).

3rd Day: Low-calorie day (same as first day).

4th Day: Moderate food day (two light meals, one protein powder meal).

5th Day: Low-calorie day (same as first day).

6th Day: Low-calorie day with food (same as second day).

7th Day: Moderate food day (same as fourth day).

Flax oil will add about 135 calories to your diet; however, that is insignificant.

Low-Calorie Foods: A Deception

It's okay to use low-calorie foods, especially diet soft drinks; but they don't help or cause weight loss.

Research has shown that low-calorie foods and low-fat or nonfat foods often have the opposite effect because people think they can just eat more. Low-fat foods are a deception that cause many people to eat more food and gain weight. Indeed, studies have shown that the fattest people use low-calorie, low-fat foods the most.

Is There a Pill?

Since most calories are burned by basal metabolism, it holds the secret to losing weight easily. Diets work because basal metabolism is usually over 1,000 calories, so even if you stayed in bed on a low-calorie diet, you'd lose weight. Therein lies the notion of a "therapeutic" approach. Think of it this way: elevate your metabolism by about 10 percent, and if you do everything the same, you'll lose 10 percent of your body weight. There are several examples.

- Smoking elevates metabolism by about 10 percent, and on average, smokers weigh about 10 percent less than nonsmokers. Conversely, smokers who quit usually gain weight even if they don't eat more to replace the gratification that smoking gives.
- Amphetamines, or "uppers" (drugs that stimulate the nervous system), are still prescribed by some doctors to help people lose and control their weight. Although uppers work because they stimulate the metabolic rate, they are not safe because they're addictive and usually cause serious mental health problems.

The herb ephedra (provides ephedrine) stimulates metabolism and is also used as a weight-loss aid. However, ephedra doesn't work for everyone, and the body adjusts (survival again); so its effect can be transient. Still, ephedrine will speed weight loss in a low-calorie diet—so you can use it to get started and then stick with the diet alone.

Recently a drug called fluoxetine has been tested on dieters. Two groups were put on the same diet; one group got a placebo pill and the other received fluoxetine. Fluoxetine elevated the body temperature by about 0.3 degrees, so those on the drug lost more weight in a given time period. More testing is required for long-term effects and safety.

Beware of Gimmicks

There are almost as many weight-loss gimmicks as there are dieters; none of them work! These ploys range from mysterious mushrooms to a special soap that removes fat, and everything you can think of in between. Each will be accompanied with a low-calorie diet—that works; the gimmick gets the credit.

Calories In, Calories Out Is Still Necessary

Even if a drug or herb is found that accelerates weight loss, people can't be on either one permanently. This means they still must manage their own calorie balance: control what and how much they eat and how much exercise they get. In short, there's no free lunch. And if there were, it would probably put weight on you.

Exercise

Exercise is an excellent approach to weight control. A fit body has more muscle, which burns more basal metabolic energy than fat. So a fit person sleeping uses more calories than does a fat person sleeping, let alone doing a day's work. Besides, exercise burns calories, so it helps get rid of extra pounds. Following is a list of routine activities that each burn about 300 calories. (In chapter 18 I have included additional exercises specifically for arthritics.)

Exercise Off 300 Calories
(Average for 150-pound Person)

Activity	Time
Brisk walk	50 minutes
Jogging (8 minutes/mile; 6 minutes/km)	30 minutes
Swimming (crawl stroke)	25 minutes
Cycling (13 miles/hour; 16 km/hour)	35 minutes

Exercise Devices

Ski machine (cross-country)	25 minutes
Rowing machine (leg and arm)	25 minutes
Stair stepper (medium resistance)	25 minutes
Stationary bike	35 minutes

A little arithmetic tells you that if you exercise at about 300 calories per day and watch your diet, you'll control about one pound every 12 days. That means that if you exercise 300 calories daily, five days a week, and cut out an equal number of food calories, you could lose a pound or more every week. So a 10-pound target loss would take a sensible 10 weeks.

However, if you exercise regularly, your 10-pound target will realistically reduce to eight pounds because you'll be building muscle, eliminating body fat, and achieving a better body size. Muscle looks better, takes up less space, and contributes to improvements in body size and shape.

Fit or Fat Is the Bottom Line

Body weight is just one indicator of fitness; more important is total body fat. Men should strive for a body weight that's about 17 percent fat, women for about 21 percent fat. Here's how to get an idea of how fit you are:

- The swimming pool test. Get in a swimming pool, curl into a ball, and exhale as you hold your head under water. If you slowly sink, you're probably about right. Sink quickly, and you're better off with even less fat. The more easily you float, the greater your excess fat.
- The mirror test. Body measurements are another approach; put on a tight bathing suit or go nude in front of the mirror and observe the following:

  With feet and knees together facing a mirror, you should see a crack of light above your knees and below your crotch.

  Find your hip bones easily at waist; go down about three inches, and you should still easily be able to touch your bones.

  Turn your side to mirror and exhale. Are your stomach and abdomen flat, and are your buttocks firm? If not, start working out regularly.
- Tape measure your hip-to-waist ratio. Measure around your hips and waist, and divide the waist measurement

by the hip measurement. The ratio for women should be 0.8 or less; for men, 0.9 or less. If the ratio is one or more, you are excessively fat and are rapidly developing heart disease.

- Hold your arm out and grip below the biceps. It should be firm and not droop. If it droops and isn't firm, you need more exercise.

On the whole, however, when ordering the focus of your efforts, your weight should come first. If you feel overweight and the scale supports your feelings, you probably need to lose weight. As you get started, take the mirror test, and then, when you have access to a pool, take the water test.

The objective is fitness—which provides a longer, more abundant life—not just to lose weight.

18

Exercise: The Miracle Drug

Exercise is synergistic. *Synergism*, from the Greek, means the sum is greater than its parts. Simply put, if you add the benefits of exercise to your diet, you get something even greater than you might expect.

Whenever you increase your activity, you also notice that your heart beats faster, which is a major objective of exercise. Think of it as nutrition, in which you are dealing with the most important of all the nutrients—oxygen. We can go without food, vitamins, and minerals for months; we can go without water for weeks, but we can go without oxygen for only a few minutes at most. It is that important.

Oxygen, similar to all nutrients, is delivered to the tissues by the blood. When you increase blood flow, you deliver nourishing oxygen more rapidly and efficiently to every tissue. As muscle tone improves from exercise, more blood capillaries develop, and the entire process becomes more proficient. Unfortunately, the converse is also true.

More important, exercise speeds delivery of oxygen and other nutrients to all the tissues, with most going to where the movement is taking place—the most active metabolism. For example, during moderate exercise, such as brisk walking, muscle temperature increases by a few degrees, which speeds metabolism in that muscle by about 30 percent.

It follows that if we flex and move our joints, this activity will increase the blood flow to them and the surrounding tissues. This promotes the healing and restoration of tissues damaged by arthritis and inactivity.

Increased blood flow also delivers more oxygen to the brain. This helps us to be more alert, overcome stress, reduce levels of anxiety and depression, and gain a better, more positive outlook. In fact, research proves that during exercise the body produces endorphins, natural mood elevators. Exercise done regularly improves the entire being—mentally and physically.

The Benefits of Flexing Joints

An old saying teaches, "If you don't use it, you lose it."

By moving and working the joints—all of them—we increase flexibility. Exercise can reduce, stop—and, in many cases, reverse—the insidious crippling that comes with rheumatoid arthritis. At the very least, exercise preserves joint mobility. The benefits can be enormous and require as little as 15 minutes twice each day—a small investment with great rewards.

Appearance

Because exercise directly involves the muscles, they benefit most from this activity. First, they increase in strength, general tone, and capacity for exercise. This, in turn, provides increased reserve capacity by helping them to become larger.

Finally, muscles are generally smooth in appearance. Consequently, as your muscle mass increases, lumpy fat disappears, and appearance generally improves.

If you increase your energy output regularly, the calories you burn will accumulate; and if you control your food intake, your weight will slowly decrease. Very often people don't really need to lose weight, they simply need to transfer the calories they store and carry around as lumpy fat into lean muscle. In the twentieth century and our land of plenty, there is no need to carry a reserve for times of scarcity.

The Benefits of More Muscle

If the appearance of increased muscle mass isn't incentive enough, the physical advantage in movement and feeling is even better. But you'll never feel the most important advantage—your increased basal metabolic rate. Think of fat as "dormant" tissue that uses an absolute minimum of the body's energy. After all, fat is storage energy, and God made it for times of scarcity so it would require only minuscule energy for maintenance. That's why a fat body has a much lower metabolic rate than a lean body.

In addition, much human fat is located just beneath the skin, where it serves as a layer of insulation. This insulating layer of fat keeps in body heat and conserves the energy required to maintain body temperature. This insulation also helps to slow the basal metabolic rate in fat people.

Conversely, lean muscle is active tissue. It is packed with blood capillaries and even stores its own energy as a carbohydrate called glycogen. Emergencies call for quick energy that muscles get from blood sugar and glycogen. Only when exercise continues for over 15 minutes do fat reserves get mobilized as an energy source.

Unexpected Benefits

Satisfaction comes with accomplishment; we all respond to positive reinforcement. You will begin to find satisfaction as you gain flexibility, shift fat to muscle, and can perform tasks you had once thought hopeless.

Mental alertness always improves because muscle tone brings improved circulation. It follows that improved circulation brings more oxygen and nourishment to your master organ—the brain.

Sleep will be sounder, not because you are tired; on the contrary, you will have more energy. You sleep better because everything about your body is more efficient. And although the restorative power of sound sleep remains a scientific mystery, no one can ever doubt its miraculous value, both mental and physical.

Regularity of bowel function will improve, another of the

synergistic benefits of exercise combined with your dietary commitment. The regularity of exercise, which tones all muscles including those of the bowel, helps them to respond easily and regularly.

Bone strength will also increase. Osteoporosis is a decline in bone density due in large part to inadequate dietary calcium and exercise in the childhood and adolescent years. Once women are past the menopause, hormonal changes bring about an acceleration of bone loss, so exercise becomes even more critical. Two factors require personal control—dietary calcium and exercise. This program will take care of the calcium, but only you can take care of the exercise!

You're Never Too Old

Careful clinical research published by Dr. Marvin Goodwin in the *Journal of the American Medical Association* has proven we're never too old to improve our health. A sampling will make my point:

Studies (since a landmark 1983 study) conducted on elderly people (65 and older) who exercised regularly have consistently yielded the same results—an increase in muscle mass, aerobic capacity, and flexibility. In addition, they had more stamina, outside interests, and greater alertness.

In three large double-blind studies, women aged 65 to 101 were given calcium supplements over a five-year period. In every case, bone density increased, fractures declined, and general health improved. These studies proved that nutrition works at any age.

When scientists evaluated what prevents heart disease in the elderly (over age 65), they learned that nutrition and exercise pay big dividends. "Good" cholesterol is the best indicator of a longer life, and this increases with exercise and a diet like the one you are following. Second, they found that, in general, lower cholesterol from a high-fiber, low-fat diet (like the one you have begun) gives longer life expectancy.

Although these studies focus on elderly people, they also prove that the earlier in life you start a healthy regimen, the better the results. Taken together, you are never too young or old to make a difference in the quality of your life.

Stretch and Breathe 15 Minutes Twice a Day

Basic limbering, stretching and breathing exercises should be done twice daily and should take less than 15 minutes each time. As you become more involved with them, don't allow that 15 minutes to decline to 10 minutes; instead, increase the amount of each.

Basic Breathing Exercises

Our objective here is to strengthen the lungs and improve on their ability to extract oxygen from the air. This is basic to our mental and physical well-being.

Abdominal breathing is best done lying down, for it requires you to hold your chest still and breathe by expanding your abdomen. Breathe in for a long five-count, and breathe out for a long five-count. Repeat this twice daily about five times or more, and you will realize that it helps you relax.

Chest breathing can be done standing; it requires expanding the rib cage on a long five-count as you breathe in and then exhaling on a long five-count. This can be practiced anytime, and should be done frequently.

Stretching and Flexing

Lower Back

Lower-back stretching is done by simply lying on your back (do this after deep breathing) and raising your knees with your hands interlocked on your abdomen. Tighten your buttocks, and pull down on your abdomen so your lower back touches the floor. Repeat this ten times.

Spinal Stretch

Kneel, with your arms on the floor, and slide your arms forward until your head just touches the floor. Keep your hips above your knees, with your toes on the floor (still kneeling). Then slide back to the original kneeling position, with your buttocks resting on your heels.

Pelvic Stretch

This exercise is difficult, but much is gained if you only try. If you keep trying you will eventually be able to do it, and that is a sure sign of progress. Lie on your back with your feet flat on the floor, knees bent. Then, with your arms flat on the floor at your sides, raise your buttocks so you shift your weight to your shoulders and feet. This should be done five times, no matter how little you can raise your buttocks.

Sit-ups

Everyone hates sit-ups, but hang in there for a few minutes. I don't care if you only start with half a sit-up. Do it! It will strengthen your back and abdominal muscles.

Lie on your back with your hands clasped behind your head and your knees bent, and sit up. If you can't make it, go as far as you can—call it a head-up. It will gradually strengthen the muscles of your back and abdomen. Aim for five, and work up to 25 over time.

Back Leg Raises

Lying on your stomach, clasp your hands behind your back. Keeping your legs straight, raise your chest and legs at the same time so your back is arched. Even if you only get your feet and head up at first, this is excellent for the back muscles and the spine. Work toward 10 daily.

Stand-up Lunge

This exercise is easy, and it's great for knees, hips, and ankles. Put your right hand on your right hip; holding your right leg in place, take a giant step with your left leg. Place your left hand on your left knee and bend as far forward as possible, holding your right foot in place and your right hand on your right hip. You'll either feel like a dancer, a fencer, an explorer, or just plain foolish.

Do this exercise at least five times for each leg. In fact, you can do it anytime you wish; it limbers knees, hips, and ankles. You see runners do it before a distance run, so it must be effective.

Knee Bends

Two types of knee bends are for us. First: sit in a straight chair. Alternately raise one leg to the horizontal and hold it for a slow five-count. Do 5 to 10 times for each leg, and each time increase a little in either time or number. You can do this one whenever you sit in a chair.

The second knee bend is easy and requires you to sit on the floor with your legs spread out. Bring your left foot on top of your right leg and pull it up with your hands as high as possible, so you're half cross-legged. Do it five times with each leg. This is excellent for the knees.

Hip Strength

Stand straight, arms at sides. Keeping legs straight and looking forward, bend to the right, keeping your arm at your side. Get your arm as low as possible down your leg. Do it five times on each side, attempting to reach the floor with your hand.

Hip Rotation

Hold something moderately heavy in your hands at waist level while standing tall. The telephone book is excellent; this book is probably too light. Now simply rotate as far to each side as possible, holding the object at each side for a slow five-count. You can do this exercise any time of the day, anywhere; it's easy, it's not strenuous, and it will do much good.

Shoulder Rotation

Place your hands on their same shoulders and raise your elbows horizontal to the level of your shoulders. Keeping your elbows horizontal, rotate them forward so that they are in front of your face. Touch elbows. Now raise your elbows over your head with your hands still on your shoulders.

Repeat this entire sequence as often as you wish, but do it

at least five times. It is another of those stretches that can be done often and at any time of day.

Now put your hands at your sides and rotate first one shoulder, then the other. Then clasp your hands in back and repeat your shoulder rotation. You cannot do this too often.

Towel Stretch

Hold a small towel (dish towel) with your left hand outstretched, and pull with the right hand. Alternate hands. While pulling, put as much strength into the pull as possible.

Then hang the towel over your left shoulder with your left hand, and grip it with your right hand reaching around your back. Pull moderately hard, left hand against right hand. Do this five times, alternating.

Hand Exercises

Arthritis is unmerciful to the hands. It can restrict their mobility to less than 10 percent and deform them even more. Don't lament over what's been lost; resolve to retain what you have and recapture flexibility that you thought was lost.

Working with hands can be very painful. Go slowly; even if you only do one-half or less at first, persevere. You will find that flexibility slowly increases with each attempt. But don't do any exercises to the point of serious pain.

Basic Hand Stretch

Stretch your hand as far as possible. If you can place your palm on the table with outstretched fingers higher than the palm, you are in excellent shape. If not, keep trying. If necessary, use the other hand to help stretch; then clench into a fist. Repeat this at least five times for each hand, and do it as often as possible throughout the day.

Finger Stretch

Touch your index finger to your thumb. If necessary, use your other hand to help as much as possible. Repeat with the second finger, and so on through the pinkie. Do it with each finger until you have a fist, then reverse the process.

Wrist Rotation

Holding your right arm above the wrist with your left hand palm down, rotate your right wrist by bringing your right hand palm up and rotate from left to right, back and forth. *Caution:* If your wrist pains when you do this, go slowly and limit your movement. If you attempt, or can complete, five at a time, you will, over the weeks, notice an increase in mobility. This is another exercise that can be done any time.

Assisted Exercise

In Chapter 26 we will explore the concept of support groups— where people get together to discuss self-help and support each other's efforts. Exercise can be a terrific activity for such groups, since any of the exercises I've discussed can be done with assistance from someone.

Assisted exercise is an excellent way to get started, especially for joints that are swollen and stiff. You must be cautious in your enthusiasm, so you don't injure someone you want to help. Start slowly and cautiously; there's no hurry. It took a long time to get your joints into this shape; it will take time to get them out.

More Vigorous Exercise

Suppose you can breeze through the exercises I've outlined. Fantastic! Do them for 15 minutes twice daily, and you are ready for more, and there's a great deal available to you.

Aerobics

The aerobics craze that is sweeping our nation is the best thing that could have happened. Some aerobics instructors conduct classes for people with restricted capability, so if there's an aerobics class in your community, see if there's a group you can enter. Sometimes, if you have a group of similarly interested friends, an instructor will hold a special session.

Vigorous Walking

Walking is an excellent exercise. It should be done in comfortable shoes, uninterrupted, with good surroundings, and in safe areas. Most important, it should be done for 30 to 40 minutes at each session. If you can walk twice daily, that is great!

Start walking short distances, and stop and rest if you are tired. Walking should be vigorous, so learn to swing your arms as you go. Breathe deeply and consistently. Do it regularly. Set aside some time each day to exercise.

The calories expended in walking range from five to about eight per minute, so 40 minutes of walking can burn from 200 to 320 calories, depending on your vigor, the terrain, and your weight. You should strive for 250 to 300 calories per session about four or five times each week; that comes to 40 minutes.

Cycling

Bicycling, at a moderate, safe cycling speed, consumes about 10 calories per minute. Therefore, 20 to 30 minutes is excellent. It builds aerobic capacity, and there is no pounding on any joints. It's got everything going for it and nothing against it.

Three-wheel bikes, now available for adults, make this activity possible at any age. In addition, it can become the transportation for shopping, errands, and socializing. It also has tremendous social value, because anyone you meet on a bicycle already shares a common interest.

Swimming

Swimming is the best exercise of all. It places no stress on joints, it uses most of the muscle groups, and it's fun. To be effective, you should strive for about 30 minutes of nonstop swimming. It need not be the fast crawl stroke shown on *Wide World of Sports*. Just keep moving, with a doggie paddle, breaststroke, backstroke, or sidestroke. If you can eventually knife through the water like a sea otter, excellent. Simply be realistic; do it regularly for about 30 minutes, and you will have achieved excellence.

Other Sports Activities

Tennis is great, but golf, as the saying goes, is a good walk spoiled. Golf is good recreation, but it is not a means of exercise. There are many recreational sports that have many merits. Think through each one to see whether it provides vigorous activity for 20 to 40 minutes. If it does, then it's excellent; if not, do it for social purposes and exercise at other times.

Mechanical Bicycles and Other Devices

Through the marvels of modern engineering you can exercise regularly in the privacy of your home. All these devices provide exercise with no jarring of joints and bones, complete safety, and convenience. With exercise devices you get what you pay for, and it's better to spend more money for one that will last.

Exercise bicycles now emphasize both the legs and the upper body. Get one where you can adjust the tension so your output can reach your capability. The advantage is that you can read, listen to the radio, or watch television while doing it. This helps to fight boredom and can make it an educational experience.

The better rowing machines allow for leg, arm, and hip activity at the same time. They increase upper-body tone a little more than the lower body, which is good, because we tend to use our legs more in daily activity.

Rowing machines use about 6 to 11 calories per minute, so 20 minutes should be the first objective, and 30 minutes the next level.

NordicTrack

In my opinion, the NordicTrack is the very best. It simulates cross-country skiing, which exercises both the upper and lower body. The NordicTrack requires a little practice to get started, but even that will help your coordination. It can be set to consume from 8 to 15 calories per minute, depending on the speed you use.

The Health Rider

Just when you think every exercise device has been invented, along comes the Health Rider. Endorsed by the health and fitness expert Covert Bailey and copied by many companies, it has several features that are difficult to beat.

Built on the simple principle of raising your own weight and distributing the effort equally between your arms and legs, it seems almost effortless. You can go as fast or slow and as high or low as you want or is appropriate; so you can gain a good workout without hurting muscles and joints.

Another compelling feature of this machine is its silence. This means you won't have to turn the TV or radio up and disturb others.

Jogging

At the risk of offending some experts, I suggest that you stop jogging. Although your arthritis might be confined to your hands, I suspect it doesn't work that way. In fact, the damage you could be doing to your knees, ankles, and toes could haunt you later on when you are older. With all the useful, nonjarring devices available today, why not move jogging into the background for occasional exercise and select a program that doesn't have the negative potential?

One Last Thought on Exercise

A great deal of research has been done on how sensible exercise can help chronic illness. Studies have proven that regular exercise improves such diverse illnesses as arthritis, high blood pressure, heart disease, and even ulcers. Other research that focuses on prevention has proven its value in preventing several types of cancer, heart disease, diabetes, and so on. In my opinion, diet and exercise are the two best tools we have to gain and maintain good health.

19

Your Chance to Control Ulcers

About 13 percent of people who have rheumatoid arthritis develop ulcers. And some medication used for arthritis, such as aspirin and steroids, actually contribute to ulcer development.

Modern medical research teaches that ulcers involve an infection, and many are successfully treated with antibiotics. However, that finding doesn't explain all ulcers, especially their prevalence in arthritics.

Prostaglandins are involved, to some extent, in helping the mucous membranes protect against excess acid. Therefore, the use of aspirin or other general inhibitors of these metabolic pathways would be an aggravating, if not causative influence. This is what is meant by side effects of drugs, and what I described in chapter 6 as the good effects of a seemingly bad prostaglandin.

Our dietary commitment should have a twofold basic beneficial effect on ulcers. It is designed to restore balance to the prostaglandins and not to eliminate even the bad one, which is good in this context. In this tug-of-war, we only want to get both sides even or give a modest edge to the beneficial. Therefore, if NSAIDs or other drugs can be reduced, the ulcer will no longer be favored or aggravated. After that, some commonsense rules and other features of this diet should apply. Any ulcer sufferer should pursue a low-fat, high-carbohydrate diet. This is logical when you recognize that a low-fat, carbohydrate-rich diet is more easily digested. It requires less production of stomach acid and helps hasten stomach emptying without an acid rebound.

What Is Acid Rebound?

Normally an empty stomach is on the acid side of neutral. When we eat food or drink a beverage, acid is produced because the food or beverage brings the stomach contents more toward neutral. If the food is not excessive in fat and contains protein and complex carbohydrates, the acid level will be restored to normal as the food digests, and the stomach will empty its contents into the small intestine for complete digestion.

Some substances we ingest, however, such as coffee, fat, and nicotine (if you're a smoker or chew tobacco), cause the stomach to overshoot its acid target and become more acidic than normal. This acid rebound—excessive acid—can overpower the neutralizing capacity of the small intestine, eventually resulting in an ulcer there. It can also help to erode the stomach lining itself and produce a stomach ulcer.

Calcium supplements are another potential aggravating factor. Select a calcium supplement made from calcium citrate; technically, that is the calcium salt of citric acid. It is not only an excellent calcium source, but it will cause no acid rebound.

In contrast, calcium carbonate, which is often used very successfully by many people, can also serve as an excellent antacid. Some people who use this acid-neutralizing calcium will develop acid rebound or even a bloated sensation, which is a somewhat similar response. If that's your experience, select the calcium citrate supplement.

The lesson is to avoid food and beverages that cause excessive acid production. The beverage of choice is tea, because it doesn't cause acid rebound and helps speed stomach emptying. Coffee, both regular and decaffeinated, should be avoided. Our dietary commitment is not rich in fat, is adequate in protein, and is rich in complex carbohydrates and fiber, all of which help produce normal acid production.

Ulcer sufferers usually produce more acid than average, and antacids are helpful to them in protecting the stomach. Antacids work on a simple principle: they neutralize the acid in the stomach. For example, a reasonable neutralizer is bicarbonate of soda—baking soda. Pour some vinegar (an acid) on some baking soda in a bowl, and watch it foam as the acid is neutralized and gas (carbon dioxide) is released. The objective is to neutralize stomach acid, but not excessively. To do this, use just enough antacid between meals, but eat enough food to keep the stomach working. Don't get in the habit of going around with an empty stomach and constantly using antacids to feel normal. Develop the habit of eating normal meals and not using acidic beverages, such as coffee and soft drinks, on an empty stomach. Drink hot or iced tea or water.

Alcohol and Ulcers

Alcohol, usually in the form of a predinner cocktail, is taken to "arouse the appetite" and get the juices flowing. Stomach juices are acid and contain digestive enzymes. If food is on its way, it's not a problem, but if the food keeps getting put off, the acid continues with nothing to digest except stomach lining. Logic tells you to eat when you drink—and the predinner cocktail should be exactly what it's meant to be—a predinner cocktail!

20

If You Have High Blood Pressure or Don't Want to Get It

If you've got high blood pressure, you're not alone. By the age of 35, 25 percent of arthritics have this problem; by age 60, 70 percent have it. Don't ignore it, do something about it!

Some of us inherit high blood pressure, and others inherit a tendency to develop high blood pressure.

Meet the Silent Killer

High blood pressure is called the silent killer because it develops so slowly that most people who get it don't know it until the doctor tells them. No one dies of high blood pressure, but its victims usually die of its complications: stroke, heart attack, or kidney failure. High blood pressure causes failing eyesight that can lead to blindness, and even a red bulbous nose and flushed face that can ruin good looks. Medication used to control high blood pressure has many unwanted side effects, and they're complicated even more by arthritis medication.

Dietary control of high blood pressure is very effective. Almost 90 percent of people with high blood pressure can reverse it and maintain control with diet alone.

Measuring Blood Pressure

Blood pressure is measured with two numbers: *diastolic,* the pressure that remains between heartbeats, and *systolic,* the pressure when the heart contracts and pushes the blood into the arteries. Systolic is normally about 40 millimeters higher than diastolic, so blood pressure is conveniently expressed as systolic over diastolic. For example, my systolic is 105 millimeters and my diastolic is 70 millimeters of mercury—more succinctly, 105/70, read as 105 over 70.

Blood pressure is expressed as millimeters of mercury because it was originally measured by how high it raised a column of mercury. The instrument used to measure blood pressure is called a sphygmomanometer. Your doctor's sphygmomanometer might use a mercury-filled column, but more modern instruments measure with an electronic, battery-operated sphygmomanometer that you can buy in many stores so as to "do it yourself." These new electronic versions give blood pressure and pulse quickly, and usually quite accurately, if the batteries are fresh. Once you know how to use one, it only takes a few minutes. Practice a few times to get it right, and be sure to keep the batteries current.

When Is Blood Pressure Too High?

When diastolic exceeds 84, be concerned. When it's regularly about 130/85, you'd better make serious dietary changes, even though that level is at the high end of normal. That is, it hasn't quite crossed over into the danger zone, but it's close, so you'd better take it seriously. At 140/90, the doctor will usually take special notice and give advice like "lose weight" and "stop using salt." He or she might even prescribe a diuretic to help lower blood pressure by eliminating salt. The statistics say we should take the warning signs seriously. At 130/85, your life will be about 10 percent shorter, on average, than someone whose blood pressure is 110/70. At 140/100 your probability of an early death is twice that of someone with normal blood pressure. Even at 130/85, it makes most other health problems worse.

The Causes of High Blood Pressure

Several dietary factors cause high blood pressure, and you can personally control each one. The odds that you can control your blood pressure by diet alone are 90 percent. If your investment odds were that good, you'd be rich beyond your wildest dreams.

Your choice of parents has an influence in cases of high blood pressure, but it isn't like blue eyes or a hooked nose. You inherit the tendency, then dietary and lifestyle factors you control (or more probably don't control) *cause* high blood pressure. Let me take you through the essential causes.

Arthritis medication can cause high blood pressure. This happens because it stops the "bad" prostaglandin that helps modulate blood pressure. The Arthritis Relief Diet will reduce your need for NSAIDs and other medication, so you can probably avoid this effect.

Salt, common sodium chloride, was once so scarce that soldiers were paid in a "salt ration," which became the word *salary.* Nowadays, we seem to live in a sea of dietary salt. The sodium in excessive salt use upsets a natural balance between two essential body elements: sodium and potassium. The other half of salt, chloride, also has a bad effect on blood pressure, especially in African-Americans, because their kidneys are more sensitive to chloride as well as sodium. That's why reducing high blood pressure by diet or medication always involves controlling salt. Most natural sodium in foods, such as milk, is different from sodium chloride, so it's relatively neutral. This natural sodium isn't as bad as added salt but must still be considered in a diet aimed at lowering high blood pressure.

K-factor is the name we give to the dietary ratio of potassium to sodium. In natural foods, the K-factor is usually three or more (three parts potassium to one part sodium). Natural diets usually have a K-factor above five, because most foods have a K-factor over 10, and many vegetables are over 100. When the K-factor falls to one (equal amounts of sodium and potassium), about 23 percent of adults and 5 percent of children will get high blood pressure. Modern diets now stand at a K-factor of 0.83. The K-factor declines from widespread use of processed foods and too much salt in home- and restaurant-cooked natural foods.

Examples of K-Factors

The K-factor is obtained by taking the ratio of potassium to sodium in food. Once you get the knack, it's easy. Table 20.1 compares some natural foods with their processed counter-parts. Notice that natural foods are low in sodium and have an excellent K-factor.

TABLE 20.1

K-factors of Some Foods

Food	Sodium (mg)	Potassium (mg)	K-Factor
Corn (one 4″ cob)	2	196	98.00
Corn flakes (1 oz.)	351	26	0.07
Canned corn (1 oz.)	251	166	0.70
Chicken (1/2 breast)	63	220	3.50
Fried chicken	1220	220	0.18
Beef (ground sirloin)	60	370	6.20
All-beef frank or sausage	461	71	0.15
Beans (2/5 cup)	3	340	113.00
Canned beans (2/5 cup)	300	264	0.90
Tuna (3.5 oz.)	40	263	6.60
Canned tuna	409	263	0.60
Nabisco Shredded Wheat	30	102	3.40
Apple (one medium)	1	159	159.00
Apple pie	282	49	0.17

Manage Your K-factor

The K-factor analysis trumpets a message loud and clear: Natural food is good news; processed food is usually bad news, unless the processor is interested in maintaining natu-ral standards, as is the case with shredded wheat in the ex-amples I gave. It is simple: eat natural foods, don't use salt in recipes, and the K-factor will take care of itself. That's what makes dietary control of high blood pressure so easy. It's healthier and costs less, so why not?

Why Not Just Take Potassium?

You've probably been thinking, "Why not take a potassium supplement to correct the K-factor and eat what I want?" It seems logical, but it won't work, because the total amount of sodium must be below about 800 milligrams daily for most people, and even lower for a few others. It doesn't matter what the K-factor is if dietary sodium is above 800 milligrams. Once you get your sodium down to 800 milligrams and eat natural food, the K-factor will take care of itself. Research has proven that there's no shortcut!

When accumulating data for my book the *High Blood Pressure Relief Diet*, I had 75 people following the dietary program. The high blood pressure of several men in the Denver area couldn't seem to budge, so I interviewed them carefully. Sure enough, one of them had a doctor friend who had prescribed potassium supplements for them; he figured they would do the job and prove me wrong. These men proved his theory was wrong—just increasing potassium alone won't do it; you've got to reduce sodium.

Read the Ingredients List

Controlling blood pressure rules out any processed food with salt on its ingredients list. Follow that rule even if the processor makes it sound okay by calling it low or moderate sodium. If salt appears on the ingredients list, don't use the product!

To continue with our list of the causes of high blood pressure:

Excess weight causes high blood pressure in two ways. First, each pound of fat contains about five miles of capillaries, small vessels through which the heart must pump blood, and it follows that the heart must use more pressure to push all that blood through those capillaries. Worse yet, the extra flab means more insulin is needed to cope with blood sugar. Excess insulin forces the kidney to elevate the blood pressure.

Both reasons lead to one simple dictum: Get your weight down!

For most, losing weight means that blood pressure returns to normal. It is the heart's way of defining upper weight limits the body can tolerate. All the experts agree, take off the extra pounds!

Insufficient calcium and magnesium will elevate blood pressure. Confirmation lies in the fact that so many people normalize blood pressure with calcium and magnesium supplements.

Fiber is essential to maintain normal blood pressure. As discussed earlier, most people only get about 50 percent of the dietary fiber they need.

Cooking to Reduce High Blood Pressure

Many recipes call for salt. The simplest of all, oatmeal (you only need to boil water), calls for salt. Don't add the salt; you'll be surprised, it tastes just fine. To enhance other recipes, you could add a drop of Tabasco sauce, seasonings, and a little white pepper or horseradish, and you've got a zesty-tasting, low-sodium food with an excellent K-factor.

How to Make Food Zesty

You can make your food taste better without adding salt. I've devised the following convenient ways to reduce added sodium to less than a few milligrams.

Four Ways to Season Food Without Salt

- *Spices.* Spices, such as "Mrs. Dash," make food tasty without any salt.
- *Horseradish.* A teaspoon of horseradish supplies six milligrams of sodium and 18 milligrams of potassium for a K-factor of three.
- *Tabasco or another "hot sauce."* A dash provides less than six milligrams of sodium and goes a long way.
- *Onions, garlic, parsley, cinnamon, and ginger.* These add zest and variety without sodium and with natural potassium.

Sandwiches: An Old Standby

Sandwiches are commonly used by all people, but most bread provides over 100 milligrams of sodium per slice and has a dismal K-factor. For example, the K-factor of rye bread is *0.3* and of white bread is *0.2.* You can solve the problem in one of two ways. In my book, the *High Blood Pressure Relief Diet*, and in low-salt cookbooks, there are recipes for excellent low-sodium breads you can make that will keep for a month or more. You can also buy low-sodium breads. For a sandwich spread, use well-ripened avocados; they have an excellent K-factor of 52, spread easily, and have fewer calories than alternative spreads. Another choice is to use horseradish with its excellent K-factor. Low-sodium, high-omega-3 spreads are also available from Spectrum Foods.

Ten Rules for Reducing High Blood Pressure

Reducing high blood pressure by diet isn't difficult. You need only the wish to take charge of your own health and destiny. In my book, the *High Blood Pressure Relief Diet*, I cover each factor in great detail; here I've summarized them in 10 rules that anyone can follow. It is less expensive to maintain normal blood pressure than to eat a diet that causes high blood pressure. So this plan has everything in its favor and nothing against it.

You've got to juggle several things simultaneously:

- *Sodium.* No complete meal should provide over 200 milligrams of sodium, and no single food should provide over 75 milligrams of sodium, unless it *is* the meal; for example, a sandwich.
- *K-factor.* Always eat for a K-factor of at least three and preferably five.
- *Weight.* Achieve and maintain your ideal weight.
- *Fiber.* Consume at least 30 grams of fiber each day. Use the fiber supplement to help. Drink 32 ounces of pure water each day; more is better.
- *Exercise.* Get 250 calories of exercise daily as described in chapter 18.

- *Alcohol.* No more than one or two glasses of wine or its equivalent daily; one is better.
- *Sugar.* Reduce added sugar to "none."
- *Fat.* Reduce fat to less than 30 percent of calories.
- *Omega-3 oils.* These oils will help to bring high blood pressure down, so this diet plan is excellent.
- *Smoking.* Absolutely never! Research has proven that smoking accelerates any inflammatory disease, especially rheumatoid arthritis.

21

Depression and Arthritis

Which came first, anxiety and depression, or arthritis? All the arthritics I know are or have been anxious about their situation, and the younger they are, the more anxious they become. Regardless of age, just thinking about their problems can cause depression.

Depression is related to serotonin, a chemical in the brain that helps you feel good. The drug Prozac, an arrow aimed at raising serotonin, relieves depression in 50 percent of users, while the remaining 50 percent improve significantly. However, Prozac is a very serious drug, and anyone should make every attempt to relieve depression without resorting to it.

Evidence is mounting that there is a relationship between hormone levels and rheumatoid arthritis. In addition, there are data to show that hormone levels reduce depression by a mechanism that doesn't involve serotonin. Research in mental issues moves slowly; however, one unexpected benefit of this diet could be a more optimistic outlook.

When Dr. Deutch and his colleagues showed that the omega-3 oils relieved PMS symptoms, including the emotional symptoms, they established the prostaglandin relationship with depression, and solid research will complete it. However, there is already much evidence that the omega-3 oils have a role in reducing depression. Omega-3 oils are consistently lower in depressed people, so there is a clear correlation that poor supplies of omega-3 oils in the diet predispose one toward depression. The same correlation has emerged in multiple sclerosis, which has many similarities to arthritis and is also characterized by depression. As you would expect, elevating the omega-3 oils helps reduce depression in these inflammatory diseases. This phenomenon also has emerged in dietary studies at the University of Oregon involving people with multiple sclerosis, postpartum depression, and alcoholism. The question for us is: "Will it help in rheumatoid arthritis?"

At this time, we do not know—and none of the dietary studies, including those where omega-3 oil supplements were used, evaluated depression or "outlook." There were anecdotal reports indicating more sound sleep, less fatigue, and a seemingly more optimistic outlook; all these conditions could be attributed to the simple fact that the arthritis improved. However, since so much evidence is mounting that the hormonal, prostaglandin, and omega-3 oil interrelationship influences mental outlook as well, that relationship probably plays a role in the depression that accompanies arthritis.

My conclusion is that this dietary program *should* reduce depression and help restore an optimistic outlook. If depression is severe enough to call for Prozac, this plan may help reduce the amount required.

Blood Sugar—Keep It Normal

Your brain responds to many changes in blood chemistry; after all, it's designed to do that for survival. The body's major source and the brain's only source of energy is the blood sugar glucose. It should be no surprise that the brain responds to a drop in blood sugar. (It also responds to elevated blood sugar, but we need not be concerned with that here.)

A drop in blood sugar can be interpreted in this way: The body is telling the brain that its source of energy is dwindling. If no obvious signs of energy are forthcoming (e.g.,

eating), the brain starts sending basic signals that show out-
wardly as anxiety. If it remains low, it could lead to a lessened
activity, even a feeling of depression.

So the first rule is to maintain normal blood sugar level.
Maintaining good consistent blood sugar also means not giving your body a *high* sugar load, because then it responds
with an overproduction of insulin. The hormone insulin
helps to get sugar into the cells to be metabolized, and an
overproduction of insulin will be followed by an excessive
decline in blood sugar. This is hypoglycemia, which means
low blood sugar. It can happen to a normal person who isn't
eating properly; it is not a disease. We should all strive to
avoid it, especially people with arthritis.

Maintaining normal blood sugar is easy—avoid a high
sugar load. Stick to complex carbohydrates, which also come
with lots of dietary fiber, and maintain a good balanced protein supply. Does that sound familiar? It should; our dietary
commitment is rich in complex carbohydrates, moderate in
fat, and adequate, if somewhat high, in protein; it all adds
up to stable blood sugar.

The second rule is to avoid large slugs of sugar. Don't eat
candy, don't use soft drinks (diet types are okay if you don't
have ulcers), and do use desserts in moderation, or select
those containing fiber, such as fruit, fruit pies, carrot cake,
and so on.

Stimulants

Caffeine is as addictive as nicotine and other narcotics. If
you drink three or more cups of coffee every day, just stop
cold turkey for two days, and you'll experience withdrawal
symptoms, albeit mild. Although caffeine withdrawal is not
as dramatic as what results from addiction to nicotine or narcotics, all the symptoms are observed by experts and felt by
the quitter. Caffeine stimulates the central nervous system,
and excessive amounts can overstimulate and produce er-
ratic activity. Have you ever heard of "coffee nerves"?

It follows that what can pick you up and add to anxiety,
can later let you down and contribute to depression. Often

fatigue has little to do with your daily work and everything to do with caffeine use. Caffeine stimulates, but when its effect wears off you feel tired. Worse yet, if you drink more caffeine to get a "pickup," you're likely to feel even more tired later on. Moderation in stimulant use is essential; one or two cups of coffee daily should be enough.

Alcohol

In the early stages of drinking alcohol, inhibitions loosen, so it acts as a stimulant and conversation catalyst. Then, as the rate of metabolism loses ground to the rate of alcohol intake, the senses begin to dull, and depression begins. All this leads to the conclusion that alcohol is a drug that should be taken seriously. It is definitely best to avoid drinking, but second best is to practice moderation—a glass of wine with a meal or a cocktail before dinner.

Nutrients, Anxiety, and Depression

The management of anxiety and depression requires good nutrition to keep blood sugar constant, plus moderation in the use of caffeine and alcohol. The metabolism of blood sugar and alcohol is dependent on such a sound nutritional foundation. This includes all the vitamins and minerals, especially the B vitamins, and the minerals zinc, magnesium, and iron.

Therefore, be sure you get enough of these to satisfy your own personal needs. You have to keep in touch with how you feel and make sure your nutritional foundation is sound. Remember, you are an individual—different from everyone else. Consequently, you might require more than your neighbor—or you might require less.

Positive Thinking

When I speak on nutrition and stress, people often ask what supplements to take for stress. I tell them that dealing with stress and the anxiety-depression spiral it produces is the same as preparing for an athletic event. We prepare for an athletic event or other performance by practicing. Nutrition is essential because it helps us to practice longer, harder, and more efficiently; it's the foundation of good health.

The situation is similar with mental health, but with a subtle difference: Mental health and stamina differ from physical health and stamina in the conditioning techniques practiced. Mental health training involves practicing outlook and meditation; they are the counterparts to physical training and relaxation. These two practices, which never fail, are best described by practitioners, as follows.

Jack (a well-known motivational expert): "My mom always taught us to be positive and find good in everything. I brought home a terrible report card; the highest grade was a C, and it had two Fs. She looked at it long and hard and finally said, 'Jack, I'm really proud of you. Any student who has trouble is tempted to cheat. I'm proud that you resisted.' "

Joanell (a single housewife, mother of four, and successful businesswoman): "Every day I sit quietly for thirty minutes, close my eyes, let my face relax, and picture a quiet mountain lake with warm sunlight. I imagine the wavelets rippling on the gravel beach and reaffirm that I'm here for a purpose and can help the world be a better place. After thirty minutes, I feel more refreshed than if I'd slept an entire night."

The best outlook was stated by Mary Kay, founder of Mary Kay Cosmetics, when chided by a newscaster for invoking religion in so many of her meetings. She said it all quite clearly:

"Why Dan, of course I call on God for help. Don't you believe you are here for a purpose? Doesn't your newscasting help people?"

I can't help you practice for stress, only you can do that. That's where the concept of a positive, motivated attitude comes in; that's the practice and you have to do it all the time.

Arthritis flare-ups always follow or accompany stress, so people who learn to see the silver lining in life's dark clouds don't let stress into their lives. Managing stress is not only important in controlling arthritis, but has even been proven to help people with terminal cancer live longer. There is no question that it works; the only issue is how successful you can make it work for you.

Raggedy Day Pick-Me-Up

(Inspiration after a flare-up or falling off the diet wagon)

- Arthritis didn't arrive in a week.
- It won't go away in a week.
- What you have accomplished is no small task.
- You will be stronger from this setback. Recall the old saying: "Whatever doesn't kill us makes us stronger."

SUGGESTIONS FOR ADDITIONAL READING AND REFERENCES FOR HEALTH-CARE PROFESSIONALS

Hibbeln, J. R., and N. Salem, Jr. Polyunsaturated fatty acids and depression, a review. 1995. *American Journal of Clinical Nutrition* 62:1–9.

22

Drug Treatment

Drug therapy for rheumatoid arthritis is frequently confusing and frustrating for the patient. The problem is that it's difficult to diagnose rheumatoid arthritis quickly and effectively.

Physicians are often criticized because of two complicating, conflicting factors. On the one hand, they usually must rely on partial diagnosis, because complete quantitative diagnosis of rheumatoid arthritis is often not possible until it's so well established that it's physically obvious. On the other hand, the course of arthritis is variable, with spontaneous remissions occurring frequently. The only scientific way to overcome these obstacles is to conduct lengthy studies on large numbers of people with rheumatoid arthritis. Such studies require large sums of money, which are always difficult to obtain. Drug companies study the disease, but the scope of their studies is oriented specifically toward individual drug therapy.

Drugs for arthritis evolved from herbal or other treatments, and this process has always been a matter of trial and error. Indeed, some herbs date back over three thousand years. For example, aspirin, the most universally effective drug, originated as dried willow bark, which was a folk remedy.

Aspirin

Willow bark as an analgesic is probably as old as humanity itself. Aspirin, acetylsalicylic acid, is found as salicylates in many other plants as well. It was synthesized (made in the laboratory) in 1855 and has been the most widely used drug for arthritis since 1899.

In 1971 Dr. J. R. Vane, a recent Nobel Prize–winner for his research on prostaglandins, demonstrated that aspirin reduced the natural production of the "bad" prostaglandin, PGE-2; this accounts for the means by which aspirin reduces the pain and inflammation of arthritis. Unfortunately, although it relieves the effects, it does not appear to slow the progress of the disease.

The Side Effects of Aspirin

Aspirin has unwanted side effects of the gastrointestinal tract. These range from mild heartburn to gastric pain and, in some people, nausea from even minor doses. Seventy percent of those who use aspirin daily to relieve arthritis inflammation will lose an excess of over two milliliters of blood daily in their stools and have a high risk of stomach and intestinal problems. Some experts claim gastric problems can be found in everyone who uses aspirin.

Animal studies have shown that the reasons are probably found in prostaglandin's protective effect on the stomach and intestinal lining. Apparently, prostaglandin PGE-2 becomes beneficial when ulcers are involved. Obviously, these observations bring to the fore the potential of a dietary approach if it can reduce aspirin or any drug use by even a small percentage.

Other side effects of aspirin include a reduction in the tendency to form internal blood clots. In fact, physicians prescribe aspirin to reduce the internal clotting in people at risk for heart attack or stroke. But this does not interfere with the normal blood clotting you would usually see if, for example, you cut a finger.

Aspirin and Vitamin C

Aspirin will suppress the growth of synovial cells cultured in the test tube or, to be scientific, *in vitro*. If vitamin C and aspirin are used together, however, much better results are obtained than from either one by itself. In science we call this a "synergistic" result. This type of research, although promising, is only helpful because even human cells *in vitro* are not a complete person.

The researchers who examined vitamin C levels in blood cells of people on aspirin therapy recognized immediately that the vitamin C levels were low and concluded that people on aspirin therapy should also take supplemental vitamin C. The same advice applies to other antiinflammatory drugs that are derivatives or analogs of aspirin.

My conclusion from this research is that if you are using aspirin or other NSAIDs (e.g., indomethacin), it is appropriate to take additional vitamin C—500 milligrams daily would probably be appropriate, and 1,000 milligrams (500 twice daily) is better. Any excess is simply eliminated.

Modern Alternatives To Aspirin—Nonsteroid Drugs

Aspirin is classified as an NSAID, but it has been so widely used for centuries that it has a special identification; so we simply call it "aspirin." Other more effective NSAIDs with fewer side effects have been developed to compete with aspirin.

At this time there are over 13 such drugs in common use, including indomethacin, sulindac, tolmetin, mefenamic acid, flufenamic acid, diclofenac, ibuprofen, naproxen, fenoprofen, phenylbutazone, azapropazon, piroxicam, and diflunisal. Others are currently being tested. Most produce results similar to aspirin, and each one has unique side effects or other actions. All have some antiinflammatory effects, but not all have been proven as effective as aspirin in treating rheumatoid arthritis. The only sure solution is careful trial and error involving patient and doctor.

Side effects on the stomach and intestine are apparently reduced with most of these new drugs; but others emerge—most notably those involving the mental status of older patients. Headaches, dizziness, an inability to concentrate, and confusion frequently signal that a return to traditional aspirin is necessary. A major advantage of these new drugs is that they have longer efficacy and do not need to be taken as often. In summary, they have some advantages over aspirin and some disadvantages; and they all work by inhibiting the body's production of the "bad" prostaglandin.

Although the NSAIDs decrease inflammation, they will not alter arthritis's course. The drugs that follow are considered "remission-inducing drugs" because their objective is to halt the gradual march toward joint destruction.

Gold

In the early 1930s, medical scientists mistakenly thought that tuberculosis and arthritis had the same infectious origins. This is understandable, because a type of arthritis often appears in people who have tuberculosis. Because gold compounds were effective against tuberculosis, doctors reasoned, couldn't they produce the same effect on arthritis? The results of gold salts on arthritis were formally reported in the medical literature of 1935. They have been used by rheumatologists ever since.

In general, gold is effective in long-term therapy for people who can tolerate its side effects. One study indicated that it slows the erosive degeneration of the joints over a period of 28 to 36 months. Other studies have shown mixed results, but in general, they indicate some clinical improvement in mobility, grip strength, and a reduction in the amount of analgesic drugs, such as aspirin, required for similar results.

Thus, gold therapy is not curative, but it reduces the progress of arthritis in the long term. In this regard, it appears to be a third line of defense and is the last-ditch effort for people who don't respond to aspirin or other nonsteroid medication.

The Side Effects of Gold

Every drug has side effects, but we use drugs because the benefits outweigh the side effects. Gold therapy has side effects that often lead to discontinued use in over 25 percent of patients. A dropout rate of over 25 percent is testimony to high, dangerous, and undesirable side effects.

These range from mild rash in over 60 percent of patients to serious kidney problems in about 2.5 percent. Complications of about 5 percent can also appear in blood chemistry, ranging from mild to very severe. For these reasons, blood and urine chemistry analyses are necessary precautions that should be taken regularly; indeed, most research physicians recommend this before each administration during the first six months of therapy and regularly, though less frequently, after that.

Gold accumulates in many of the major organs, including the liver, kidneys, and spleen. Although this is not surprising, it undoubtedly imposes metabolic stress on the body. Thus the maintenance of sound nutritional status is imperative. The Arthritis Relief Diet and its basic supplement plan should be excellent for that purpose.

Gold has no known interactions with nutrients; therefore, this dietary plan and supplement use should not interfere with gold therapy, or vice versa. Indeed, this diet is so nutritionally sound it should be supportive, reducing both the level and duration of therapy.

Penicillamine

Penicillamine decreases the immune complexes in rheumatoid arthritis. It appears to be similar to gold in efficacy and would be the fourth line of defense. Clinical results indicate that it reduces swelling, the RF, the number of joints involved, and the subjective pain that develops.

The Side Effects of Penicillamine

About 50 percent of patients who start penicillamine therapy can still continue after one year. It has side effects similar to gold therapy, ranging from mild rash (44 percent of patients) to serious blood and kidney problems in a few individuals. It also appears to induce an autoimmune syndrome in some people. This is a serious concern to any physician, and is thus carefully monitored.

One side effect is that hypogeusia—taste perception—is dulled. Although this usually passes in about three months, appetite loss usually accompanies it because food has no taste or tastes like chalk. This is a good reason for people on penicillamine to follow a sound diet and supplement plan.

The Nutritional Effects of Penicillamine

Penicillamine is a chelating agent that interferes with metal absorption (e.g., iron). Therefore, to prevent iron or other metal deficiency, penicillamine should be taken about one and a half hours after meals. It should not be used at the same time that supplements containing minerals are used. In fact, because supplements should be taken with meals, it would be best to delay the use of penicillamine for one and a half to two hours. It is helpful to double up on the basic supplement plan.

Steroids

The injection of corticosteroids into an arthritic joint often brings remarkable relief. An oral steroid medication is also available. Unfortunately, the relief is not always sustained, so steroid therapy is useful only as support for other forms of therapy. For example, low-dose, oral steroid administration is sometimes used as an adjunct to other drug therapies to relieve symptoms while the drugs are beginning to take effect; or steroid injection is administered to relieve severe symptoms.

The dramatic relief from steroid use appears to be strictly symptomatic—that is, it relieves the symptoms but has no effect on the underlying disease. This relief, however, is so dramatic that there is a tendency to increase the dosage to gain further relief, and as this is done, the side effects begin to become more obvious.

Side effects of steroid use range from skin ailments to seizures, and many adverse reactions in between. None of them are trivial—like a rash that goes away—so physicians use steroids with great caution.

Nutritional interactions have not been clearly identified. The chronic use of steroids produces so many side effects, however, that the patient must maintain a good nutritional program. Not only should this dietary commitment be maintained, but additional supplements are certainly desirable.

Cancer Chemotherapies and Immunosuppressive Drugs

Drugs that suppress the immune system should, in principle, be effective against rheumatoid arthritis. Most of the drugs used (e.g., methotrexate) are chemotherapeutic agents effective in reducing malignancies. Put another way, this is cancer chemotherapy applied to arthritis.

Although some success has been observed, no drugs have been studied in detail and in large enough numbers to know the extent of their effectiveness. In general, the side effects and toxicities of these powerful agents could be much more serious than simple rheumatoid arthritis itself. These drugs are generally used where all else has failed or is no longer effective. This means that at this time, these drugs are the last-ditch effort!

Nutritional Effects

Methotrexate, the most widely used cancer chemotherapy drug, interferes with a B vitamin, folic acid. Therefore, for the drug to be effective, supplements should not be used within eight hours of taking methotrexate. This allows ample time for the drug to be absorbed and the body to eliminate the excess.

In the use of all these powerful agents, loss of appetite is a common side effect. Consequently, the Arthritis Relief Diet should be followed, and supplements should be used to maintain a higher-than-average nutritional status. Doubling of the supplement could be a basis of insuring your basic nutrition.

Reflections on Drug Therapy

Pharmaceutical science is making great strides in treating arthritis from a scientific approach now that the biochemistry of inflammation and joint damage is understood, as opposed to a strictly empirical approach. Without doubt, this progress will bring new and far more effective drug therapy with minimal side effects.

At this time, however, I cannot help but be concerned that some of the existing therapy (e.g., gold shots continued for 10 years or more) might be worse than the disease itself. But the American approach to illness has traditionally been through medication and the entire system—medical education through insurance—supports it.

It is very confusing: Why do authoritative agencies and physicians themselves often reject out of hand the possibility that diet can have a significant effect on supporting drug therapy? In a journal they will report treatment of 27 people with a drug, and if only a few have some success—albeit minor—the drug will get extensive recognition. In contrast, the notion that diet can help to restore balance to the prostaglandins and optimize drug therapy gets rejected out of hand, in spite of clinical studies on large numbers of people. More important, the diet program recommended here can only do good and no harm.

Indeed, the side effects of some drugs can be so devastating that in the long term they shorten life and reduce its quality. Therefore, if a dietary commitment has any chance of reducing drug use, it should be as welcome as a cool breeze on a hot day.

Reducing Drug Use

A physician's objective is to cure his or her patient. In most cases that is exactly what happens, but arthritis is different because it is always there—sometimes in remission, sometimes flaring up. Thus the doctor's objective, by necessity, shifts to keeping it minimized.

Placed in the context of drug therapy, this diet plan will help your body produce a balance between the antagonistic and beneficial prostaglandins. In published clinical studies, this approach has already reduced inflammation and pain, on average, by 70 percent in specific cases. Therefore, a reduction of drug use should be possible; in some cases it can be reduced to zero!

The reduction of the medication requires collaboration between the patient and physician. One thing is certain: Only you know how you feel; your doctor must take your word on that. In addition, he or she would like to see you reduce your drug intake as much as possible, and so will be pulling for you as well. Your doctor can precisely evaluate chemical and physical changes but relies on you to explain how you feel. You should insist on one thing: that he or she be positive. Tell your doctor, if it is needed, that you don't want to hear this "diet can't do anything" talk.

23

Herbs

Throughout time, people have cultivated physiologically active plants to relieve, cure, and prevent illness. The *Codex Ebers*, an Egyptian papyrus written about three thousand six hundred years ago, listed over four hundred plant-based remedies for many common illnesses. Interestingly, garlic was the most often used herb among them. One thousand years after *Codex Ebers*, in ancient Greece, Hippocrates, the father of modern medicine, also used plants to cure and prevent many illnesses. In fact, some of his remedies are still used.

Every medical history of Asia, Europe, the Americas, and the South Seas confirms that special plants, commonly called herbs, were used to treat illnesses.

Some people argue that any useful plant is an herb, but that would make carrots or cabbage herbs, because they can be used to cure night blindness and soothe ulcers, respectively. A more practical definition limits the use of the term "herb" to situations when a plant is used therapeutically. For example, garlic cloves sliced into spaghetti sauce, as food, make the difference between a plate of spaghetti and a pasta experience. Yet as an herb, garlic can stop infection and save lives, reduce blood pressure, and—correctly worn around the neck—ward off vampires and colds; yes, the people about whom the vampire myth developed had an extreme sensitivity and a violent aversion to garlic. These people suffered from porphyria, a disease characterized by severe light sensitivity and very painful reactions to the active chemicals in garlic. Hence they avoided both light and garlic. This genetic disease developed in the European areas where the vampire legends abound.

Intuition tells us that arthritis, which has always afflicted people, has led to the use of many therapeutic herbs. In fact, any modern herbalist or book on herbs will offer many herbal remedies. I have included a description of the herbs that have apparently stood the test of time. Since few, if any, double-blind clinical studies have been conducted, the only recourse is to select those herbs that have withstood the trial and error of hundreds, if not thousands, of years.

Feverfew (*Tanacetum Parthenium*)

Feverfew is also known as *Chrysanthemum parthenium*; its leaves have been widely used for headaches, migraine headaches, and arthritis. These three illnesses have some common inflammatory characteristics.

In migraine, and sometimes in other headaches, the inflammation of membranes in the head squeezes down on blood vessels, restricting blood flow to certain areas of the brain. In contrast, when a vessel itself inflames, blood flow often increases since its diameter expands. In either case, inflammation is involved.

Feverfew was used so widely for migraine headaches that it was clinically tested in the late 1970s and 1980s. When correct care was taken in preparation, feverfew leaves not only relieved ongoing migraines, but regular daily use prevented or at least reduced the severity of subsequent migraine headaches. In fact, discussions with migraine sufferers who used feverfew always revealed that if the headaches didn't stop, they were never as bad. So we can confidently conclude that feverfew has withstood double-blind testing for an inflammatory illness, migraine headaches. It's reasonable to expect that feverfew's folk use for arthritis will similarly stand up to clinical testing, if it is ever conducted.

Scientists have concluded that the physiologically active

components in feverfew inhibit the enzyme system that produces the bad prostaglandin PGE-2, the very same one we explored in chapter 6. It's also possible that feverfew's active chemicals work at a level different from other antiinflammatory drugs. Perhaps their best attribute is that they don't *stop* production of the "good" prostaglandin, PGE-3, and its companion leukotriene.

Folk wisdom reports that feverfew not only relieves inflammation but also works on pain. In addition, these observations suggest that it stops the production of the bad leukotriene. Since feverfew is also used to reduce severe cold and flu symptoms, there's little doubt that its mechanism of action focuses on the prostaglandin system—specifically, the bad, not the good one.

However, where there's good news, there's usually a caution or even bad news. Some active components of feverfew, the parthenolides, are easily destroyed by heat and exposure to air. This short "shelf life" explains why some people who use and swear by feverfew regularly say it doesn't always work. That's another way of saying, "Not every batch is good." Therefore, if you decide to try feverfew, be sure that the active components are listed, or that the person who sells it can represent its potency.

Feverfew is completely safe when used correctly; however, used to excess, it can cause diarrhea. So don't take it with the idea that "if a little is good, more is better"; be sensible, consult an expert, and work up to an effective use.

Question: If I follow this diet, can I still use feverfew?
Answer: Absolutely yes!

Wild Yam (*Dioscorea Villosa*)

Wild yam is also known as colic root and rheumatism root, the latter term supporting the folk wisdom that this plant helps arthritis. The active components are stored in the rhizome, which contains many active steroids and steroidal saponins. These materials, as mentioned earlier, help accelerate the removal of the bile wastes, which seem to aggravate arthritis. The traditional use of wild yam to promote bile output and thus relieve the discomfort of gallstones is a secondary clue to the effectiveness of the saponins.

Wild yam has been widely used for rheumatoid arthritis and the more common osteoarthritis. Herbalists have prescribed wild yam, probably for centuries, to counter the acute inflammatory phase of arthritis. Similarly, it apparently has an ability to make a headache less intense. Hence, it probably has some components resembling those found in feverfew.

In 1943, Dr. Russell Marker produced two kilograms of the female hormone progesterone from the wild yam; until about 1970, the wild yam was used to make the birth-control pill for women. This supports its other folk use, which was to relieve menstrual cramps. It's just one more clue that some of its active components can suppress production of the "bad" prostaglandin.

If you are following the Arthritis Relief Diet and wish to experiment with wild yam, sensible use should be completely safe.

Devil's Claw (*Harpogophytum Procumbens*)

The active part of devil's claw is a tuber used by herbalists. Its major use is in arthritis.

Devil's claw has been studied and shown to have antiinflammatory properties. Research done in Germany, and more recently in France, suggests that devil's claw has antiinflammatory and pain-stemming effects similar to cortisone, a pretty powerful modern drug. However, these studies are at best preliminary, and follow-up studies are needed to quantify the results. Therefore, take comparisons to cortisone cautiously and consult with an expert herbalist regarding the use of devil's claw for arthritis.

Black Cohosh (*Cimicifuga Racemosa*)

Also called black snakeroot, bugbane, and squawroot, black cohosh is a North American herb that is used for headaches, high blood pressure, and the easing of muscle cramps; and both the dried root and rhizome have been used as folk remedies for premenstrual cramps.

In reading herbal literature and consulting herbalists, one gets the impression that black cohosh has two things going for its use on arthritis: salicylates and muscle-relaxing effects.

Aspirin is a salicylate, has antiinflammatory properties and probably works by the same mechanism. The second effect, the dilation of blood vessels to increase blood flow, will similarly reduce the muscle pain often associated with arthritis.

Bogbean (*Menyanthes Trifoliata*)

Bogbean, as you might have surmised, grows in marshes and bogs; both leaves and rhizomes are used.

Bogbean is another herb that provides a generous supply of saponins, the fiber also obtained from alfalfa (which is a much better source). In my opinion, however, saponins are not the source of bogbean's effectiveness, because the amount of bogbean normally used would not supply enough saponin to be consequential.

Although I have no solid evidence, I believe that bogbean is probably a reasonably good source of the omega-3 oil alpha linolenic acid. When it is used regularly in ample quantity, it would definitely bring a modest level of relief.

Indirect confirmation of my hypothesis stems from the historical evidence that bogbean helps relieve "rheumatism," the term often used to describe mild rheumatoid arthritis, which often flares up when the weather goes from warm and mild to cold and damp, signaling that a low-pressure system has moved into the area.

Sarsaparilla (*Smilax Officianalis*)

Once sarsaparilla root was used to flavor soft drinks, and many people over age 50 probably remember sarsaparilla soda. Herbalists now use the root to treat arthritis and psoriasis, a variant of arthritis. There is no scientific evidence of its effectiveness.

It is interesting to note that sarsaparilla root was a sixteenth-century cure for syphilis that persisted up to the twentieth century, even though there is not one scintilla of evidence to support its effectiveness.

Conclusions About Herbs

As the curtain is descending on the twentieth century, we are witness to a revival in the use of natural materials, especially for healing. Indeed, this diet is a natural dietary approach to help keep arthritis in check, or to reduce it to such a low level that your life can be abundant. Similarly, the five herbs discussed here can help. In researching them I didn't come across any unwanted side effects. In fact, to the contrary, people reputed, especially about feverfew, that they generally felt better and even more optimistic.

Their use for hundreds, if not thousands, of years is strong evidence that herbs provide some level of relief. My only caution is to be sensible and make your errors on the side of safety.

Let me hear of your results.

Quackery

Arthritis is especially susceptible to quackery because its flare-ups are usually unpredictable in their onset and duration. It follows that if some treatment is applied while the flare-up is occurring, both the designer of the treatment and the afflicted victim conclude that the treatment works. If the inflammation and pain subside (go into remission), the purveyor of the treatment has yet another follower, if not disciple, to sell the cure. If the attack recurs quickly, the victim usually seeks a different treatment or one that is currently in vogue.

Many studies worldwide have proven that between 50 and 70 percent of arthritis patients seek "alternative treatment," which usually means a special diet (not the plan in this book), copper bracelets, or some other device, as well as the use of special dietary supplements. This general trend seems to prevail in the United States, England, Australia, Japan, and most European countries.

Surveys by the University of Toledo on people with arthritis have revealed the following: Over 40 percent say diets have helped them achieve relief, about 21 percent say vitamins bring relief, and 8 percent benefits from copper bracelets. There are no reports on the effects of either acupuncture or homeopathic treatments, which are also widely used.

Because arthritis is a joint disease, the treatments often

take on some external, physical application, such as a "field force" or some other sophisticated-sounding application of electronics. Indeed, history teaches that arthritis treatment is rife with "creative" applications. Most of these are variations of the simple application of heat, which brings temporary relief to the joint. This is especially true if the flare-up has been brought on by change in the weather. But these treatments have no relationship to diet, and I simply want you to beware of them and recognize that they don't really work.

Pills, nostrums, and elixirs have been sold to arthritics for as long as we know. In fact, the most commonly prescribed drug—aspirin—first appeared as willow bark, which was and has always been our most effective cure-all. Diet has often been attempted, prescribed, and even scientifically tested, and finally we now know why some relief has been realized.

The simplest diet is to starve oneself, possibly taking only water and fruit juice. It usually worked for arthritics, and today we know that this was because it removed the source of arachidonic acid and sensitivity. It reduced the tendency to produce the "bad" prostaglandins.

Similar conclusions can be drawn about vegetarian diets, which have prevailed for hundreds, if not thousands, of years, and have a wide following. But even this approach has often been branded as quackery because there was no long-term testing. In hindsight, we know it probably helped, but the diet was not complete enough because it didn't provide sufficient omega-3 oils. The Arthritis Relief Diet goes about as far as we can in using commonly available foods and sensible food supplements.

Another level of pills and nostrums, that goes beyond diet, purport either to cure or bring relief to arthritics. They consist of ingredients ranging from snake venom to extracts of exotic clams. Snake venom sounds dangerous, and clam extract, although probably harmless, could have an offensive odor. But even if the use of such materials is not inherently dangerous, it is harmful because it diverts the sufferer from treatment that can help—and that is quackery.

Copper Bracelets: A Folk Remedy Reconsidered

Copper salts (ionic copper) inhibit the biosynthesis of prostaglandin PGE-2, which, as you know, causes inflammation. This is well established, and the metabolic systems involved are well characterized. In fact, they appear to work similarly to gold salts in this respect.

Copper bracelets have been used by arthritics as a form of folk medicine for decades—if not centuries. This practice has been branded quackery by the government, the Arthritis Foundation, health columnists, and me! Briefly, everyone jumped on the bandwagon declaring "fraud!" All that occurred before research began to uncover the relationship between the prostaglandins and inflammation. Indeed, some medical scientists still speak of the prostaglandins as though there is only one.

Copper bracelets interact with some people's perspiration to dissolve significant amounts of copper, some of which penetrates the skin in some people by the process of percutaneous absorption and enters the circulatory system. Although studies comparing copper bracelets with aluminum bracelets suggest that copper does help relieve the inflammation, the matter clearly warrants further study, because there are much more effective means of getting copper ions to the inflammatory site than by the use of a bracelet. Until more research is conducted, copper bracelets cannot do any harm, and in spite of their previous branding as quackery, they might benefit some people. I'm keeping a skeptical but open mind.

Sometimes There Is Another Side to the Story

Copper bracelets always turn up when quackery is discussed. Although I don't advocate their use, one research physician explained it as follows:

> The enzyme (cyclooxygenase), which makes prostaglandin PGE-2, is inhibited by copper ions. Some people who use copper bracelets get enough copper by percutaneous absorption (absorption through the

skin) to elevate blood levels and inhibit the enzyme. Comparison to aluminum bracelets has proven that there is a small number of people who are helped by copper bracelets. (Peter E. Gray, M.D., verbal communication)

Although Dr. Gray's comments sound reasonable, scientific evidence is definitely wanting. Nevertheless, copper bracelets have been used for hundreds of years. When folk wisdom stands the test of time, it deserves critical analysis.

Common Sense Should Prevail

Although I've said it already, I'll say it again: Arthritis is not curable in the sense that an infection can be cured with antibiotics, or an illness—like measles—can be either prevented by vaccination or allowed to just run its course. In contrast, once arthritis is established, even if it seemingly clears up completely, the potential for recurrence remains.

Therefore, any simple device, pill, or nostrum that purports to "cure" should be avoided, unless you can be shown the kind of proof that is documented in this book.

Getting It All Together: People Helping People

25

Mental Conditioning

Michelangelo, asked how he could create such beautiful sculpture from mere pieces of stone, replied that the statue was in the stone; all he did was chip away the residue. He visualized the statue, sketched it, and then maintained that vision as he carefully eliminated the excess.

So it is with life. You've got to visualize what you want to become—visualize yourself achieving that goal. If an objective is realistic, even if it is a stretch for you, it can be achieved. Gaining control over your arthritis is not different from any other objective.

Is the Glass Half Full or Half Empty?

Identical twin boys were born to a couple whom experts agreed should never have lived together, let alone had children. The boys' father, an unskilled worker, never held a steady job; he lived from day to day and had no goals. When the mother could get work, she did menial tasks. Both parents drank excessively and often lived on welfare. The boys were raised as much by neighbors and each other as by their parents. By the age of 10, they were almost completely on their own.

Survival was the word that described their home life.

Their parents fought so violently at times that the police were called to stop the argument, and they slept off their alcoholic condition at the police station. Both parents often beat the children and used words like "damn kids" or "no-good kids." This home life did not spawn a healthy outlook.

By the age of 35, the twin boys were a study in contrast. Tom was an unskilled worker, didn't hold jobs very long, drank heavily like his parents, and fought with his wife. He and his wife lived in the same squalid environment in which he had been reared. They were well known to the welfare authorities and learned to take advantage of everything the government would provide.

Jim was the complete opposite. He had worked hard at menial part-time jobs while going to school at night and on weekends. He saved what little money he could, and when he finished school, he started a small business. By the time he was 35, Jim's small company was growing, and he was becoming a wealthy man. His family life was also rewarding. He and his lovely wife worked together with their two children in a harmonious atmosphere. Their modest home was neat and clean and expressed pride of ownership. They were a close, happy family; they enjoyed life and were optimistic about their future.

A social worker doing a study about identical twins interviewed both brothers. She asked each the same questions, so as not to bias the study. Curiously, she got exactly the same answer to one pertinent question: "Why did you become what you are today?" The answer was: "What else could I do growing up in that place?"

Each man had exactly the same lack of opportunity, but each had a different vision of himself. Tom saw himself as nothing. Jim saw himself as anything he wanted to become, with no place to go but up. The only difference between the brothers was how they got from where they were to where they visualized themselves. For Tom, it was easy—do nothing. For Jim, it required commitment to an objective. Tom said to himself: "This is what life is like." Jim said to himself: "I can always do better than this."

Success Begins with Goals

When I began working on this diet I found myself involved with two groups of people: those who wanted to transfer responsibility to others and those who wanted to take responsibility for themselves. More important, I could see the former become the latter if they were able to reduce this diet to daily tasks. They learned that success was within themselves if they proceeded one step at a time toward a realistic, clearly defined goal.

The Bag Story

A rather heavy woman approached me at a meeting and asked if this diet would relieve the pain in her knees. Realizing that the diet would definitely help if by nothing else than losing weight, I said, "Only if you will make a commitment to losing ten pounds." She immediately replied that she simply couldn't lose weight, because diets never worked for her. I told her this diet would—if she would only give it a chance and monitor her progress with a fat bag. I explained that the fat bag is simply a cloth sack that she could buy or make. Then I instructed her to purchase a 10-pound bag of gravel from an aquarium or garden supply store. Each time she lost a pound she should add a pound of gravel to the cloth sack, which she should put in a prominent place and carry with her whenever she ate out. Within five weeks she had lost 10 pounds and was working on another 10! She bought another bag—the first one was in the family trophy case!

The fat bag externalized her daily goal of losing weight and transferred this major objective into a simple symbolic task—filling the bag. The arthritis pain diminished from both the weight loss and the food changes. She enjoyed newly earned freedom and mobility and an exhilaration she had forgotten since she was a young girl.

Set an objective, reduce it to some daily tasks, and you will succeed!

A Simple System that Works

Objectives work best when we are constantly reminded of them. It follows, then, that we've got to use the facilities—and people—available to remind us. I have a simple system that works for me; I'll explain it for you.

Write your objectives and goals clearly on 3 × 5 note cards. Keep one set attached to the refrigerator with magnets. Recruit your loved ones, especially your children, to help. Keeping your objectives spelled out where everyone can see them will maintain their support. It works!

Carry a set of objective cards with you so you are reminded that we want this plan to become habit. Place one more set on your dresser or wherever you get ready in the morning and evening so you'll see them first thing and last thing each day.

Sound corny? It's not.

What's corny is the notion that you could have a chronic disease and not use every resource at your disposal to improve the health you've got, and reduce the illness to its absolute minimum. In that light, simple note cards are monuments to human willpower and positive mental attitude.

Objective Setting for Arthritis

Your broad objective can be simply stated: "Maximize personal control over arthritis." Notice this doesn't include or exclude doctors, diet, medicine, exercise, or anything. It simply states that you want to have as much control over this illness as possible. This broad objective should be reduced to daily tasks, which control each variable at your disposal. We have already explored each one—diet, medication, exercise—and when you finish this chapter, you'll have a start on mental outlook.

Diet is the first line of control most of us have over our health. Indeed, when Hippocrates said "Let food be thy medicine," he recognized the control it can have over our health. Unfortunately, most people allow that responsibility to be taken by other people—mother, spouse, friends—and it takes willpower to get it back. Set some food-related objectives that are so clear you can't miss. That way you will regain control.

Goal I: Find Your Flare Points

If you're fortunate enough to be able to control flare-ups through food, you're a lucky person indeed, because you're in control. Most of the people who follow this diet plan have identified foods that cause their arthritis to flare up. The more systematically they approach their quest, the more successful they are. You've got to keep the food diary. If you eat the wrong thing, your joints usually respond within 12 hours.

Goal I: Keep a food diary and find your flare foods. Once they're found, you're in control.

Goal II: Make this Diet Become Habit

While we've talked about diet all through this book, you must still put it into effect *"one bite at a time."* Reducing it to daily menus is all that is required. And depending on your circumstances, this means planning food one day at a time.

You're the controller, and you must use your resources effectively. The best way is to plan each day the evening before. In this way you will do two things automatically: plan your food and food supplements, and take control of your time.

Use your food diary to write down what you plan to do the next day. At the end of that day you can simply write a report card on how you did—and how you feel—and then what you're going to do the next day.

Goal III: Weight Control

Get your weight under control. If you're not overweight, think "exercise" to firm up; then read on, because you're going to start helping others and you'll need some preparation.

Once you decide to lose weight, write down your goal

clearly in pounds and inches, and *use a fat bag* to monitor progress. By using the food diary, willpower, and the fat bag, you'll reach your goal. Once you get good results, and if you're typical, you'll want to go further and lose more; but remember, one pound at a time.

Goal IV: Stress Control

I'm often asked, "What should I take to control stress?" I can detect the stress in the voice even if it's over a telephone. My heart goes out to the person at the other end, because I want to give a simple answer, and I can't. Controlling stress requires conditioning for stress. The next question I get is, "How do you condition for stress?"

Conditioning for stress is no different from the way athletes train for an event; only the practice for stress is mental instead of the physical practice required for an athletic objective.

Positive Thinking

Mental conditioning can be practiced all day, every day. This is in contrast to physical conditioning, which requires special equipment, time, and other restrictions. Mental conditioning requires much more self-discipline, however. Positive thinking, positive mental attitude, positive recognition, and positive action are all involved. Let's explore how each of these helps.

In each situation you must first apply the maxim that something positive exists in every situation; then find it; and then build on it; don't dwell on the negative. Nancy, a 45-year-old woman who was one of the original 50 women who followed this plan, spoke to me once with a beautiful example; the conversation went like this:

"Dr. Scala, I've got a flare-up like I haven't had in months." I immediately started to console her. "No," she immediately responded. "I'm glad; you see, we went to a party last night and since being on your diet, I haven't had chopped liver." I nodded in agreement as she continued. "This flare-up proves a point; I know that I shouldn't eat chopped liver and drink so much wine."

Positive Outlook

A positive outlook is faith in the concept that the future will always have opportunities to do good and be better. People who start this plan have a positive outlook even if they don't recognize it. They have faith in themselves that they can take control of their health and things will improve.

Positive Mental Attitude

A positive mental attitude is a little more subtle. It requires searching for the silver lining in the cloud that's on the horizon. It is an attitude that the future is always a little brighter than the present. It's the attitude that allows people to see beyond their condition and build for a brighter future.

Positive Recognition

Positive recognition is the easiest of all. You only have to say something nice to someone. Suppose it's a waitress. Before you place your order, say "What a nice smile you've got," or "That color is very becoming," or "You have beautiful eyes." The idea is simple: Find some way to recognize something good in your fellow humans. This recognition will come back to you many times over; you'll find good things in yourself.

Positive Action

Last is action. You need to love yourself, and there's no better way than by doing something positive anonymously. Help a stranger, give an anonymous gift, leave a bundle of clothes for someone in need. But also do it so people know you do it. If someone does something well, give him a "thumbs up" sign. A "thumbs up" is easy. It could be as simple as this note: "Dear Kim, I'm proud of your work, and how you remembered Mom's birthday with that beautiful card."

Think of how you'd feel if you got one! If you start now, you'll be surprised how effectively these actions condition your positive mental processes. You'll need it—because you've got an illness that won't quit; stress that won't quit. The only way to beat stress is to maintain mental conditioning the same way a world-class athlete maintains physical conditioning.

26

Shoulders to Lean On: Support Groups

People need people. Explore how arthritics can help arthritics. New methods of treatment are constantly emerging, such as this dietary plan, and self-help groups.

I asked one woman what was the most memorable thing she learned at her arthritis group meeting. It was the side effects of the penicillamine therapy her physician was using. He had mentioned the side effects, but she hadn't heard him—for any number of reasons, probably nervousness; but when she mentioned how she felt to the group, another woman told her what to expect and how long it would last and helped her learn to cope.

Even so, there is much more to derive from groups than just helpful hints. Possibly the most helpful outcome is the positive thinking we just explored. You will see how other people cope and realize that no matter how difficult things may seem, there are other people who are worse; you can be thankful that you have the health you do. When you go to an arthritis help group, try to learn from other's experiences and help them by sharing what you have learned. You will discover much by listening to what causes flare-ups and how to avoid them. All the foods and variations that fit into this dietary plan would take volumes to write down, so discussing them is beneficial. If you start a group just to talk about dietary issues, there is no end to the meetings and discussions you can have. But there's more.

Medical Knowledge

The Arthritis Foundation publishes excellent literature on your illness; and they have chapters of their organization in many areas and will be happy to serve as the catalyst for discussion.

Physicians who specialize in arthritis—and no matter where you live, there is one in your area—are flattered by invitations to speak. They can explain the methods of medication, the side effects, and why one course of therapy is chosen over another. They can also learn from you—yes, they will never know your illness like you do—and the subtleties of the causes of flare-ups will help them with other patients.

I have spoken to many arthritis discussion groups and have learned more from them than they from me. Sure, I tell them all about prostaglandins, EPA, and diet, and I discuss the history of arthritis and other interesting things. However, their questions give me valuable information about their day-to-day arthritis concerns. As Confucius said, "To teach is to learn," and a good teacher always learns more than his students.

Help Others

The most important benefit of an arthritis support group is what you can do for others. I have the advantage of speaking all over the world, and I meet people with every type of ailment imaginable. Very few seem as desperate or frightened as the young women who have just learned they have arthritis. You can do so much to make these people learn that they can cope, help their physician gain control, lead a productive life, raise a family, laugh, and have fun. You can set an example with your own positive thinking, optimistic outlook, and support. You can send them a "thumbs up."

Group support does even more. There are times when the inflammation and the pain reduce the outlook to an all-time low. These are the times when people want to quit, and that is when they need maximum support; they need someone to carry them with mental support, to visualize the sunshine over a dark horizon.

Peripheral Support Speakers

This plan emphasizes diet, so dietitians would make good speakers for arthritis support groups, as well as excellent counselors. But don't stop there; invite exercise physiologists, therapists, chiropractors who work with arthritics, and others. Furthermore, these specialists should be able to discuss the benefits of various types and levels of exercise for differing arthritic conditions.

Dietitians who take this commitment seriously can speak and help design menus and foods that meet all the criteria. But don't invite dietitians who are unwilling to look beyond the basic food groups, or who deny the need for basic supplementation. Supplementation is fundamental to your way of life.

Nurses who work with rheumatologists are informative speakers and often the unsung heroes of modern medicine. They usually have more time to observe the subtleties of arthritis than does the physician. Their ability and willingness to explain self-help is endless. A little recognition of them will go a long way.

Clothing specialists who make garments that are less restricting and help ease sensitivity should also be invited. These people can learn much from you that will accrue to their economic advantage; so once more your efforts will reach others.

Pharmacists can talk about the medications that are most frequently used—and abused—and those that are most current. More important, the pharmacist can alert you to drug interactions.

27

Personal Stories

I want you to see yourself in this chapter. Many people have helped in the development of this plan, and I have gotten to know them personally. From this interaction, several characteristics about arthritis have emerged that helped me to understand both the illness and the people it affects.

After many discussions, I have concluded that stress and arthritis go together.

The medical approach is unclear. Drugs help a great deal, but I'm confused about gold shots and wonder if, after being on them for 10 years, the cure creates more problems than the illness.

Diet is undoubtedly effective in helping to relieve inflammation, and specific foods clearly cause flare-ups in some people but not others. It is neither an allergy nor a food sensitivity in the classic sense. An allergy usually causes a rash or some similarly obvious reaction, while a sensitivity usually causes upset, diarrhea, or both.

Weight loss helps by removing a serious stress on joints; moreover, it imparts a renewed self-image. Self-image, like positive thinking, can make life with a chronic illness more bearable.

Exercise emerges as an elixir that cannot be discounted. People who find the means to exercise can't praise it enough. Even the most restricted people can do some form of exercise.

I hope you will enjoy the following lessons from personal experience as much as I have.

(I have not used peoples' real names. They were kind enough to share their experiences with me so that others may benefit, and I respect their anonymity.)

Stress, the Starting Point

Adults who get arthritis can usually trace its beginnings to some specific event, such as childbirth; but there are many others. Men have usually traced their arthritis to some sports injury. Very often it's a knee that was injured in baseball or football. But often the arthritis starts later in life, and with some type of stress—usually in the form of an illness.

Linda's Story—Childbirth

Linda has three children and has been taking weekly gold injections for five years. She is finding the Arthritis Relief Diet helpful.

> *Dear Dr. Scala:*
>
> *My arthritis just appeared after I had my first baby. At first the doctor wasn't sure but he took some tests and told me. My knees had swollen and my wrists hurt.*
>
> *While I was carrying my other two children I felt wonderful. There wasn't a hint of the problem. I never ached or even felt stiff.*
>
> *After my second child I was so bad that I had to stay in the hospital a week. Everything ached and I felt terrible.*

Linda went on to tell me that she wished she could be pregnant all the time without having children. As she put it, when she was pregnant she felt great. After her third child her arthritis progressively worsened.

Betty's Story—An Accident

Betty is faithful to the Arthritis Relief Diet plan, and the benefits she has derived are gratifying. The way in which her arthritis appeared is typical:

> *I had to drop a cake off at church and I left my car without putting the brake on. It started rolling so I put the cake down and ran to stop it. I slipped on the ice and was pinned between my car and another car. My right knee was very badly bruised.*
>
> *I spent a week in the hospital and then a week at home before I could go back to work. At the end of the week in the hospital, my wrist started hurting. While at home it continued to bother me and became swollen, so I asked the doctor to look at it. He thought it was from work, the way I opened and wrapped packages. At the end of my first week at home, the week after the accident, my ankle started hurting and it was swollen. It got red and sore!*

With sore and swollen ankle and wrist, her doctor tested for arthritis. Sure enough, Betty tested positive. Yet she could always control the inflammation and pain with standard oral medication, even though she couldn't continue working.

Nancy's Story—An Accident

Nancy has arthritis in her right leg, shoulder, elbow, and wrist, and the middle and index fingers of her right hand. It started about 25 years ago when her right side was injured in an auto accident. After she left the hospital, she noticed that when she woke up, the middle finger of her right hand would ache—not a sharp pain—an ache. It progressed to her wrist, elbow and shoulder. Now it's in her spine and right leg. She relates that it took about two years to spread.

Nancy has used both alfalfa supplements and this diet to rid herself of the pain of arthritis. She sticks to the diet and takes medication only when necessary.

Leslie's Story—Stress of Divorce

Leslie is 35 years old, has five children, and was in excellent health until her husband asked for a divorce. Right after the divorce she noticed that she would wake up with pain in both hands and shoulders. When the pain was accompanied by swelling (about four months later), she went to the doctor.

She was diagnosed with arthritis. Slowly she progressed through the drugs and eventually was put on oral gold and cortisone.

Leslie has regressed to a poor condition; it has affected her hands, toes, shoulders, and knees. Her muscles are bad, and now her jaw has become involved.

As evidence of the continuing stress, she is unable to sleep and is so often tired she cannot get up in the morning. This stress spiral, I have come to believe, is typical; arthritis feeds on itself. The illness can be so devastating that it creates fear of what is happening, the future looks bleak, the medication makes you miserable, and the stress gets worse. As the stress progresses, so does the medication. It can become a vicious spiral that only goes down.

Since my first book on arthritis, Leslie has doggedly followed the diet plan and only needs a nonsteroidal anti-inflammatory drug occasionally. She has remarried and, as the old saying goes, is living "happily ever after."

Beth's Story—The Affair

Beth developed arthritis following the stress of a serious marital problem. She met an old flame while visiting with her mother, and one thing led to another—call it biology. Her arthritis coincided with her extramarital affair and the conflict she had with her rigid Catholic upbringing.

Guilt can be a terrible stress on the body and cause anyone to become run-down. In Beth's case, the exhilaration of finding herself still desirable was finally overcome by the guilt and near destruction of her marriage. It was devastating! But all is fine now; her marriage is sound, and she has the arthritis under control.

In contrast to Leslie, because Beth took control and stopped the stress, or for other reasons, the progression of the arthritis stopped. She got along on aspirin (or a little stronger medication) until she started the diet. Now she's off everything!

Ruth's Story—Willpower

Ruth had arthritis for several years and finally realized that the spiral of anxiety, depression, and sleeplessness was destroying her. She decided that was all she would tolerate. From that day on, her arthritis has not gotten any worse; and with this diet and her doctor's help, she is getting better. She sleeps well, eats well, and exercises regularly.

Connie's Story—It Just Came

At 16, Connie woke up one morning to discover that she felt terrible and she couldn't get up or walk. The arthritis traveled from her knees to her hands and wrists. Wrist rotation froze within a month. The next step was gold shots—and they helped. In her own words, "I could tell when it was time for the shots because I hurt so."

Connie and I could find no stress other than normal high-school activities. About one year before the onset of arthritis, however, she was so tired she would go to bed as soon as she arrived home from school, and sleep until the next morning, with a short break for dinner. This went on for weeks; her doctor tested for mononucleosis and a thyroid problem. Neither test was positive, and she eventually came out of it.

In hindsight, the fatigue should have been pursued further, because she had always been such an active person. Such a dramatic change in activity was surely symptomatic of an illness.

Stress—Some Conclusions

Without attempting to practice medicine or to diagnose, I can draw some conclusions. It appears to me that stress is a type of trigger for arthritis. Most of the women I have spoken to could trace the beginnings to a stressful event, either physical or emotional; usually it was some of both.

Working with athletes makes me respect mental power, and I now believe that stress can go both ways. Guilt and other forms of emotional stress can be such a drain on the body's reserves that a disease can start. And if the researchers who trace arthritis to a virus are correct, emotional stress can reduce the immune capacity enough to allow this illness to take hold.

Injury does the same thing, but it's more obvious in that case that the body's reserves are challenged and that the arthritis has won.

Food Diary Results

On a recent TV talk show a physician showed film clips to illustrate how food sensitivities aggravated arthritis. The physician injected an extract of certain foods into selected patients. The results were dramatic. Within hours joints would swell and become immobile, and pain was written all over the volunteers' faces. The doctor made his point in vivid, living color.

Unfortunately—or fortunately—most sensitivities are not that clear. Moreover, most of us can't afford to have food extracts prepared and tested by capsules or injections. Experience with the personal discoveries people have made using food diaries show that the situation is not as clear and well defined as the doctor's dramatic illustrations.

Elizabeth's Story—Milk and Eggs

Elizabeth keeps a food diary, and it didn't take long for her to discover that dairy products—milk, yogurt, and most cheeses—will bring on swelling, pain, and reduced mobility of her knees, ankles, and wrists. But her experience with eggs is interesting.

"If I eat two eggs three days in a row, on the third day I can feel the flare-up coming. By the fourth day I can hardly get out of bed." She continued, "I ate a poached egg once when my niece stayed with me, and felt fine. With a little experimenting I learned that I can tolerate an egg now and then. It's only when I have more than one at a time, or one every day, that I have the problem."

Elizabeth asked the salient question: "Dr. Scala, can that be correct; could I tolerate one egg from time to time? Or could it all be in my head?"

I told her it isn't in her head; after all, she carefully evaluated her response to certain foods. She got in touch with her body and knows its limits. Whatever it is in eggs that causes the flare-up, she simply must not exceed her threshold level.

Alice's Story—Tomatoes

Alice and her husband live in the Midwest. The diet worked very well for her. In her own words: "I feel so much better with my arthritis I can hardly believe it. I have always heard you are what you eat; now I believe it. Thanks to you, and to my daughter who took the time to send me your diet."

Alice kept a food diary, and by trial and flare-up learned that she cannot eat tomatoes. She can, however, eat potatoes and eggplant. She confirms my notion that the nightshade plants should not categorically be eliminated. Alice stays closely with the plan and uses the food diary; she has not identified any other foods that cause trouble.

Patricia's Discovery—Mocha Mix

Patricia cannot use dairy products, even skim milk; she found that it produces inflammation. However, in her own words: "I agree on the advantages of oatmeal. One way to enjoy it for breakfast is to use an artificial nondairy creamer such as Mocha Mix, which is found in the dairy section."

Bernette's Story

Bernette has followed the diet faithfully; she cannot eat grapefruit and tomatoes. "I found I was not able to eat grapefruit, as my knees and elbows became sore. Last summer when our tomatoes were producing, I foolishly ate a lot and my joints became very sore. When I stopped eating tomatoes, the pain and swelling went away. I found since following your diet that my ankles are not puffy at night as they have been for a long time."

It's quite clear that Bernette reacts to certain foods. Most interesting, none of them fall into a pattern—grapefruit and tomatoes are quite different. The disappearance of ankle puffiness is similar to what other people and physicians report.

Losing Weight

Sometimes I feel that I've found the ideal weight-loss diet. Everyone who's started the Arthritis Relief Diet did so for arthritis, but every letter or telephone conversation includes a statement about losing weight.

Barb's Story

Barb is a registered nurse who started some friends on the diet. She used two of them as examples to get other people to her arthritis support group, and provides us with two excellent testimonials:

Phyllis' story—as told by Barb—tells how well she feels: reduced pain, and then, after four weeks, "There is less cloudiness in her eyes; happily she has lost five pounds."

Frances's story—as told by Barb—explains how well she is doing; for example, in less than a week she felt improvement in her knees, but the weight loss came at the end. "Frances also is losing unwanted pounds at a rate of two pounds a week, and who wouldn't feel good about that?"

Rusty's Story

Let Rusty tell it in her own words: "Since beginning the arthritis diet, my weight has gone from 165 pounds to 145 pounds. That's okay, as I'm 5'9" tall and never was heavy until arthritis limited my activity. I've also taken three to four inches off my waist! That's terrific!"

Obviously, the plan works effectively as a weight-loss diet and, as Rusty put it so clearly, helps to shift the weight; measurement, not pounds, are what count. Rusty has ankylosing spondylitis, and she has found much relief from this diet.

Exercise

Most people try to exercise, and it becomes very difficult as the arthritis worsens. But one woman, Thelma, described something so beautiful that I feel it should be shared.

"I go to the municipal indoor pool to exercise."

I quizzed her further: "Do they have a program there?"

She replied, "Oh, heavens no. I get into the water and do the exercises you told me to do. In the water it doesn't hurt; I guess it keeps the weight off my knees."

I was surprised, so I asked if she does it alone.

"Oh, no, I have lots of friends now, and we all do it. Some of them have to get in up to their neck because they aren't as good as me; but they are seeing results."

I can't tell you how gratifying it is to see people helping people like that. And the common sense that led them to do it is astounding. So I asked Thelma if it helped.

"Well," she said, "look at it this way—I used to get a ride to the pool because I couldn't walk that far, and now I walk both ways."

General Results

Many people have now followed this plan, and I'll share some short comments in addition to those already expressed.

Lydia: "I feel I am doing something right now; the signs of arthritis have disappeared."

Elsie: "I am on your arthritis program and have improved quite a lot."

Donna: "I am feeling so much better; I should have written sooner."

Alice: "I feel so much better, I can hardly believe it."

Elmer (age 81): "I started it April ninth and haven't seen any improvement. I'll stick with it for three more weeks." In three weeks I spoke to Elmer. "I'm starting to see results; I notice I can get right up in the morning now."

Carol (age 31): "I can't tell you how great it feels to be normal again. I am just astonished." (She goes on to explain what she can't eat.) "I don't have a tinge of pain, no soreness. I feel great."

Ursula (reporting on her mother): "We are afraid to be overly optimistic, but she had almost immediate results. As of today, her leg and foot are normal, all swelling gone. Her hands look normal; the swelling is gone."

Yvette: "I've been following your diet for a month now, and I've noticed a big difference. I'm not as stiff, and I have more strength. I feel very good and have dreams of walking without any more problems."

Joyce: "I felt good on the diet to begin with, so I don't feel better. I have found that when I have any forbidden foods I experience a flare-up, usually within eight hours or less—most often in my wrists or hands. I do believe that by following this diet plan the quality of life for many people would improve."

Connie: "I feel great, because now I'm doing something positive and the diet works. My doctor will work with me to spread out the gold shots. I've been on them for ten years and would like to reduce them."

Conclusions

I could go on and on with testimonials. They indicate to me that people gain improvement in their lives and more freedom from the flare-ups that seem so common. If people will only use a food diary, and start with the *Do's* and *Don'ts*, the quality of their lives will improve.

All this has confirmed one very important teaching for me. We are personally responsible for the food we choose, and we cannot escape the observation that we are what we eat.

First Year Anniversary

Assess how you feel.
Are you faithful to your diet?
Are you able to dine out successfully?
Does the food diary keep you on track?
Are you enjoying life more?
Are you sharing your good fortune?

Keep up the good work!

AUTHOR'S COMMENT:

Working on this book has been fulfilling. After all, who wouldn't enjoy sharing important new scientific findings with people to help them keep their disease under control and inspire them to live a life with more quality?

I would like to hear from the people who use this book. Let me know your experiences, what you've learned, and how it has helped you. Write to me at:

44 Los Arabis Circle
Lafayette, CA 94549

Index